GEORGE T. LIU, DPM, FACFAS
Associate Professor, Department of Orthopaedic Surgery, The University of Texas Southwestern Medical Center, Foot and Ankle Service, Orthopaedic Surgery, Parkland Memorial Hospital, Level 1 Trauma Center, Dallas, Texas

ANDREW J. MEYR, DPM
Director, Temple University Podiatric Surgery Residency, Clinical Associate Professor, Department of Surgery, Temple University School of Podiatric Medicine, Philadelphia, Pennsylvania

JOHN MILLER, DPM
Resident PGY-2, Baltimore VA Health System, Rubin Institute for Advanced Orthopedics, Baltimore, Maryland

ORHAN K. OZ, MD, PhD
Department of Radiology, The University of Texas Southwestern Medical Center, Dallas, Texas

VIRGINIA E. PARKS, DPM, AACFAS
Department of Surgery, Division of Plastic and Reconstructive Surgery, Hospital of the University of Pennsylvania, Philadelphia, Pennsylvania

KEVIN RAGOTHAMAN, DPM
Department of Plastic and Reconstructive Surgery, Center for Wound Healing, MedStar Georgetown University Hospital, Resident Physician, Division of Podiatric Surgery, MedStar Washington Hospital Center, MedStar Georgetown University Hospital, Washington, DC

KATHERINE M. RASPOVIC, DPM, FACFAS
Assistant Professor, Department of Orthopaedic Surgery, The University of Texas Southwestern Medical Center, Foot and Ankle Service, Orthopaedic Surgery, Parkland Memorial Hospital, Level 1 Trauma Center, Dallas, Texas

DREW T. SANDERS, MD
Assistant Professor, Department of Orthopaedic Surgery, The University of Texas Southwestern Medical Center, Orthopaedic Trauma Service, Parkland Memorial Hospital, Level 1 Trauma Center, Dallas, Texas

CARLOS H. SEREZANI, PhD
Assistant Professor, Division of Infectious Diseases, Departments of Medicine, and Pathology, Microbiology and Immunology, Vanderbilt University Medical Center, Nashville, Tennessee

MICHAEL CYRUS SIAH, MD
Department of Vascular Surgery, MedStar Washington Hospital Center, Washington, DC

JOHN S. STEINBERG, DPM, FACFAS
Professor, Department of Plastic and Reconstructive Surgery, Co-Director, Center for Wound Healing, MedStar Georgetown University Hospital, Washington, DC

JENNIFER C. VAN, DPM
Faculty, Temple University Podiatric Surgery Residency, Clinical Assistant Professor and Chairperson, Department of Surgery, Temple University School of Podiatric Medicine, Philadelphia, Pennsylvania

MICHAEL VAN PELT, DPM, FACFAS
Associate Professor, Department of Orthopaedic Surgery, The University of Texas
Southwestern Medical Center, Dallas, Texas

ELLIOT WALTERS, MD
Department of Plastic and Reconstructive Surgery, Research Fellow, Center for Wound
Healing, MedStar Georgetown University Hospital, Washington, DC

STEPHANIE C. WU, DPM, MSc, FACFAS
Associate Dean of Research, Professor, Department of Podiatric Surgery and Applied
Biomechanics, Professor, Center for Stem Cell and Regenerative Medicine, Director,
Center for Lower Extremity Ambulatory Research (CLEAR), Dr. William M. Scholl College
of Podiatric Medicine at Rosalind Franklin University of Medicine and Science, North
Chicago, Illinois

DANE K. WUKICH, MD
Professor, Chair, Department of Orthopaedic Surgery, Department of Internal Medicine,
The University of Texas Southwestern Medical Center, Foot and Ankle Service,
Orthopaedic Surgery, Parkland Memorial Hospital, Level 1 Trauma Center, Dallas, Texas

JACOB WYNES, DPM, MS, CWS, FACFAS
Fellowship Director, Limb Preservation and Deformity Correction Fellowship, Assistant
Professor, Department of Orthopaedics, Co-Director, UMMC Limb Preservation Clinic,
University of Maryland, University of Maryland School of Medicine, Baltimore, Maryland

Contents

Diabetes prevalence is increasing in the United States. As of 2017, 30.3 million people in the United States have diabetes (9.4% of population). Of these, an estimated 7.2 million persons are undiagnosed. Prediabetes, a condition that is associated with peripheral neuropathy and is a precurser to diabetes, affects 83.1 million or 33.9% of adults in the United States. Diabetes is most commonly diagnosed by fasting plasma glucose or by an A1C test. An oral glucose tolerance test can also be used, but its use is primarily restricted to research settings.

Diabetes mellitus is an international epidemic. In the United States, the prevalence of diabetes has increased from estimates in 1990 when 6.5% of the population was affected and 6.2 million people had diabetes compared with the estimates in 2017 with 24.7 million people with diabetes or accounting 9.6% of the adult population. The diabetic foot syndrome manifests as a combination of diabetes-related diseases including diabetic sensory neuropathy, limited joint mobility, immunopathy, peripheral arterial disease, foot ulceration, and Charcot arthropathy. The culmination of these provides an ideal environment for unrecognized tissue injury that leads to ulceration, infection, infection, and amputation.

The accurate assessment of peripheral perfusion is a critical step in caring for a diabetic patient with active ulceration. This article guides the provider through diagnostic and therapeutic options. The perfusion assessment begins with a physical examination and augmented using noninvasive tests. Although some of these tests can be performed at the bedside, often a dedicated vascular laboratory is required. Additional cross-sectional imaging studies or formal angiography should be performed as well. These tools aid in the creation of the best therapeutic plan, which aims to restore perfusion and allow for rapid wound healing via open or endovascular means.

The etiology of ulcerations in diabetes mellitus is associated with the presence of peripheral sensory neuropathy and repetitive trauma due to normal walking activities to areas on the foot that are subject to moderate or high pressures and shear. The combination of loss of protective sensation, deformity, and repetitive trauma is the perfect storm for ulcer development. Once an ulcer is developed, the most important part of the healing process is offloading the ulcer site. Offloading is the mainstay of healing neuropathic ulcers.

early intervention, and prophylactic procedures, most surgical interventions for this condition are reactionary. Patients still primarily present to emergency departments with acute infections and tissue necrosis. The surgical intervention for this results in soft tissue deficit, often with partial foot amputation, through excisional debridement of pathologic tissue. Minimizing this initial soft tissue loss, with subsequent reconstruction of the defect, forms the focus of this article with a detailed anatomic assessment of structures at risk in the forefoot, midfoot and rearfoot.

Tissue defects that result from diabetic foot infections are often complex and necessitate reconstructive soft-tissue surgery to achieve closure. Intrinsic muscle flaps of the foot require attention to major vascular pedicles and are useful for closing smaller ulcerations. Microvascular free flaps are beneficial for large defects and provide long-term survivability. Perioperative planning is an important aspect of caring for diabetic patients requiring reconstructive surgery. These techniques are valuable tools for use in efforts to preserve a functional limb in this patient population.

Surgical bone reconstructive procedures of the foot and ankle in diabetic patients must be considered when performing evaluation of a diabetic foot for patients with preulcerative lesions and preexisting wounds. Preventive deformity correction can reduce the potential risk of ulceration, infection, and possible amputation in a patient with an at-risk foot type. It can also expedite wound healing and prevent further breakdown in a patient with lower extremity ulcerations. This article discusses different types of surgical bone reconstructive procedures as preventive and prophylactic deformity corrections to reduce osseous deformity, minimize preulcerative lesions, and increase limb-salvage rates in the compromised patient.

Reconstruction of the diabetic Charcot foot can be a challenge even for the most experienced foot and ankle surgeon. The first portion of this article discusses the preoperative evaluation with an emphasis on factors that can be modified before surgical reconstruction to help optimize surgical results. The second portion of the article focuses on intraoperative methods and techniques to help improve postoperative outcomes. Surgeons should strive to provide high-quality, cost-effective care by optimizing patient selection and perioperative care. Objective measures of patient outcomes will become increasingly important with the transition from volume-based to value-based care.

Amputations distal to the ankle joint are commonly performed in efforts to
preserve a limb. Thorough examination of lower extremity biomechanics,
patient functional status, and patient goals must be used to help prevent
reulceration and further amputation. Once infection is resolved in the acute
setting, musculotendon balancing should be considered at the time of
amputation closure to maintain functionality of the limb. Patients should
be closely followed postoperatively and monitored for biomechanical
deformity that needs to be addressed. Careful attention to detail and
adherence to surgical principles can help keep patients active and prevent
further amputation.

Poorly controlled diabetes with comorbid manifestations negatively affects outcomes in lower extremity trauma, increasing the risk of short-
term and long-term complications. Management strategies of patients
with diabetes that experience lower extremity trauma should also include
perioperative management of hyperglycemia to reduce adverse and
serious adverse events.

Patients with severe diabetic foot ulcerations that fail to heal with standard
conventional therapies may be candidates for hyperbaric oxygen therapy;
these patients also should be evaluated for atypical wound etiologies.
Medical evaluation includes thorough history, physical examination,
screening laboratory tests, and ulcer biopsy. During hyperbaric oxygen
therapy, patients breathe 100% oxygen at 2 times to 3 times atmospheric
pressure while enclosed in a hyperbaric chamber. Over time, administration of hyperbaric oxygen therapy can result in wound neovascularization
and enhanced limb salvage. In patients with suspected atypical ulceration,
referral to a multidisciplinary wound healing center is considered standard
of care.

CLINICS IN PODIATRIC MEDICINE AND SURGERY

SERIES OF RELATED INTEREST

Foot and Ankle Clinics
Available at: www.foot.theclinics.com
Orthopedic Clinics
Available at: www.orthopedic.theclinics.com

THE CLINICS ARE AVAILABLE ONLINE!
Access your subscription at:
www.theclinics.com

Preface

Diabetes and its Impact on the Lower Extremity

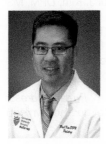

Paul J. Kim, DPM, MS
Editor

I am grateful to participate in this *Clinics in Podiatric Medicine and Surgery* dedicated to Diabetes. It is my hope that the readers gain important insight that will translate into better care for their patients. The following series of articles cover a variety of topics that attempt to provide some degree of clarity for the care of the complex diabetic patient. The authors were selected based on their reputation and depth of understanding about this disease and its manifestations in the lower extremity.

It is important to acknowledge that diabetes is a systemic disease that deleteriously impacts every organ system in the body. Its manifestation in the lower extremity, most commonly the diabetic foot ulcer, is simply a sign that reflects this relentless disease process. Although our understanding has increased with evolving science regarding its pathogenesis as well as increasing number of treatment options with the advent of novel therapies, too often the disease overwhelms the host, and our treatments result in failure.

It is important to better understand the host. This is best described in the equation below:

$$\text{Healing Potential} = \cfrac{1}{\cfrac{\text{Bacteria} \times \text{Perfusion} \times \text{Tissue Mechanics}}{(\text{Host})^{X}}}$$

$$X = \text{Unknown}$$

Healing potential is driven by the denominator. Some of the variables can be impacted, including bacteria, perfusion, and biomechanics. However, healing potential ultimately is dependent on the host. The host can be defined by multiple, perhaps innumerable variables. This includes genomics, comorbidities, nutrition, and socioeconomic

Clin Podiatr Med Surg 36 (2019) xiii–xiv
https://doi.org/10.1016/j.cpm.2019.03.003
0891-8422/19/© 2019 Published by Elsevier Inc.

status. This variable is then multiplied by an unknown exponential. Until we truly understand the host, there is little hope for sustained healing.

Perhaps our goals should be adjusted to focus on things like prevention, reducing recidivism, and most importantly, improving the quality of life for our patients. The topics throughout this issue provide invaluable information for the care of the diabetic patient.

Paul J. Kim, DPM, MS
Medstar Georgetown University Hospital
Center for Wound Healing
1st Floor Bles Building
3800 Reservoir Road Northwest
Washington, DC 20007, USA

E-mail address:
Paul.j.kim@gunet.georgetown.edu

Medical Management of the Diabetic Patient

Stephen Clement, MD

KEYWORDS

• Diabetes • Medical management • A1C • Insulin

KEY POINTS

• Both surgeons and clinicians must adjust to the growing epidemic of diabetes.
• The investment of time and energy for surgeons and clinicians to partner with each other will provide dividends in better surgical outcomes and healthier patients.
• Good glycemic control will lead to better surgical outcomes.

EPIDEMIOLOGY

Diabetes prevalence is increasing in the United States. As of 2017, 30.3 million people in the United States have diabetes (9.4% of population). Of these, an estimated 7.2 million persons are undiagnosed. Prediabetes, a condition that is associated with peripheral neuropathy and is a precurser to diabetes, affects 83.1 million or 33.9% of adults in the United States.[1]

HOW IS DIABETES DIAGNOSED?

Diabetes is most commonly diagnosed by fasting plasma glucose or by an A1C test (**Box 1**, from American Diabetes Association [ADA] Standards of Care).[2] An oral glucose tolerance test can also be used, but its use is primarily restricted to research settings. Patients with classic symptoms of hyperglycemia and a random glucose level greater than or equal to 200 mg/dL have diabetes (see **Box 1**).

WHAT IS "BORDERLINE DIABETES?"

Patients are unfortunately told by their care providers that their diabetes is "borderline" or they have a "touch of sugar." This terminology is a falsehood and should be discouraged, because there are specific guidelines for diagnosing diabetes as discussed earlier. Labeling their diabetes as "borderline" suggests that the condition is not serious, resulting in the patient being complacent about the diagnosis. For example,

Disclosure Statement: The author has nothing to disclose.
Endocrinology, Department of Medicine, INOVA Fairfax Hospital, 3300 Gallows Road, Falls Church, VA 22042, USA
E-mail address: Stephen.Clement@inova.org

Box 1
Criteria for the diagnosis of diabetes mellitus (any single criteria is sufficient)

Fasting plasma glucose ≥126 mg/dL.[a]

Two-hour plasma glucose ≥200 mg/dL during an oral glucose tolerance test, using a glucose load containing 75 g anhydrous glucose dissolved in water[a]

A1C ≥6.5%[a]

In a patient with classic symptoms of hyperglycemia or hyperglycemic crisis, a random plasma glucose ≥200 mg/dL

[a] In the absence of unequivocal hyperglycemia, results should be confirmed by repeat testing.

From American Diabetes Association. 2. Classification and diagnosis of diabetes: Standards of medical care in diabetes-2018. Diabetes Care 2018;41(Suppl 1):S15; with permission.

---

the OB/GYN physician does not tell their patient that she is borderline pregnant. Patients with the diagnosis of diabetes should be told so and urgently referred for diabetes education and treatment.

TYPE 1 VERSUS TYPE 2

The vast majority of nonpregnant patients with diabetes are classified as type 1 or type 2 diabetes. The older terminology of "juvenile onset" or "adult onset" has been abandoned, because type 1 diabetes can occur at any age and children can develop type 2 diabetes. Currently, there are no well-established criteria for determining this classification other than good clinical follow-up. In general, patients with type 1 diabetes require insulin from an early age and will quickly develop ketoacidosis if insulin is not taken. In contrast, patients with type 2 diabetes frequently need insulin, but they can also be well managed with a variety of noninsulin replacement medications, as well as diet and exercise. In addition to type 1 and type 2, women may develop diabetes in pregnancy. There are also several rare forms of monogenic diabetes or diabetes associated with other conditions (ie, cystic fibrosis, acromegaly, Cushing syndrome, steroid associated diabetes).

WHAT IS GOOD DIABETES CONTROL?

Good diabetes control means adequate control of the plasma glucose, as well as other major cardiovascular risk factors such as blood pressure and cholesterol, considered together as the ABCs of diabetes care (*A*1C, *B*lood Pressure, *C*holesterol). Large randomized studies for both type 1 diabetes and type 2 diabetes have shown that good glycemic control reduces risk for microvascular complications. The target A1C based on these pivotal studies is less than or equal to 7%.[3] This target is recommended for the patients who have a long life expectancy and who are motivated to reliably follow the regimen prescribed. As will be seen in the following sections, diabetes therapy can be complex and adherence to a complex regimen difficult. For this reason, patients who have advanced complications or who may not have a long life expectancy may best be served with a higher A1C target. The target A1C that is realistic for the patient should be a joint decision between the patient's physician and the patient.

IS MEDICAL MANAGEMENT COST-EFFECTIVE?

Medical management as described earlier requires frequent office visits and use of multiple medications. Ortegon and colleagues[4] performed an economic model to determine the cost-effectiveness of optimal foot care (ie, protective foot care, education, regular inspections of the feet, identification of the high-risk patient, treatment of nonulcerative lesions, multidisciplinary approach to foot ulcers) versus optimal diabetes care. For each intervention, the investigators calculated the incremental cost for each quality-adjusted life-years (QALYs) saved for the 2 interventions. They found that both optimal glucose control and optimal foot care reduce lower extremity amputations and that the 2 interventions are additive, as the cost per QALY saved is reduced in patients who receive both optimal glucose control and optimal foot care (**Table 1**).

WHAT IS PATIENT-CENTERED GLYCEMIC MANAGEMENT?

Patient-centered glycemic management is tailoring the therapy to the patient's goals and his or her ability to carry out the plan, as well as factoring the practical aspect of being able to afford the diabetes medications and supplies. The first step is to conduct a comprehensive evaluation of the patient's personal characteristics (ie, level of motivation, comorbidities, and cultural beliefs) as well as their personal goals for care, access to medications, and concern over cost of medications and supplies. Once these are assessed, the physician and the patient agree on the management plan that is measurable and achievable. The next steps in the cycle are monitoring the efficacy of the plan and trouble-shooting snags in plan implementation, followed by plan revision. During the process, the provider must keep in mind that 100% of diabetes care is self-management. The patient must "own" the plan. The role of the care provider is to facilitate and guide the patient in their lifelong journey of self-management.[5]

DIABETES SELF-MANAGEMENT EDUCATION AND SUPPORT

Diabetes self-management education and support (DSMES) is the new term of what was previously known as diabetes education. The goal of DSMES is to provide the instruction so that the patient can make informed decisions and take ownership of his or her diabetes. DSEMES is most commonly provided in face to face sessions with a diabetes educator, either individually or in groups. The ADA provides Recognition for programs that fulfill a strict set of requirements for providing quality education (see URL). The programs exist as free-standing centers, hospital-based centers, and within private practice offices. The ADA maintains a list of listing or recognized programs.[6]

WHAT IS THE ROLE OF DIET AND EXERCISE?

As the growth of obesity in the population is the primary driver of the diabetes epidemic, attention to lifestyle behaviors is crucial to successfully managing the disease. The dietary plan should be individualized to the patient with the help of a registered dietician who is experienced is working with patients with diabetes. Many patients are attracted to "Fad" diets that may result in initial weight loss, but over

Table 1 Cost-effectiveness of glucose control versus optimal foot care	
Treatment	Cost (Thousands per QALYs Saved)
Optimal Foot Care	$23
Optimal Glucose Control	$32
Optimal Foot care and Glucose Control	$12

the long term are not healthy or not sustainable. If the patient is overweight, the dietitian works with the patient to achieve measurable goals of weight loss while maintaining healthy amounts of food types and without sacrificing goals for other targets such as blood glucose and blood pressure. This patient-focused counseling is called medical nutrition therapy.[7]

Current exercise guidelines recommend that patients with diabetes should engage in 150 minutes or more of moderate to vigorous intensity aerobic exercise per week, spread over at least 3 days per week.[7] Because patients lose their mobility with foot and lower extremity problems, they commonly have extreme difficulty reaching these aggressive goals. Limited mobility commonly starts a vicious cycle that leads to worsened diabetes control and higher risk for additional complications. This underscores the importance of maintaining mobility through aggressive limb preservation, good podiatric care, and physical/occupational therapy.

DIABETES MEDICATIONS

Diabetes research over the past 20 years has produced many new classes of medications that have benefits over older medications. The practice of choosing the appropriate medication and the sequence of adding medications have kept clinicians, professional associations, and journal editors busy. The most current medication guideline was recently published.[5] The guideline highlights 2 classes of medications, the glucagon-like receptor agonists (GLP-1 RA) and the sodium-glucose cotransporter-2 inhibitors, which are now preferred over other diabetes medications for patients with cardiovascular disease. A list of each class of medication is listed in **Table 2**.

Table 2
Commonly used noninsulin diabetes medications

Drug Class	Agents	Medication Type	Generic Available	Worrisome or Common Adverse Effects
Biguanide	Metformin	Pill	Yes	Diarrhea
DPP-4 Inhibitors	Alogliptin Linagliptin Saxagliptin Sitagliptin Vildagliptin	Pill	No	None
Sulfonylureas	Glipizide Glyburide Glimepiride	Pill	Yes	Hypoglycemia
SGLT-2 Inhibitors	Canagliflozin Dapagliflozin Empagliflozin Ertugliflozin	Pill	No	Urinary tract infection Ketoacidosis
Thiazolidinediones	Pioglitazone Rosiglitazone	Pill	Yes	Weight gain Fluid retention
GLP-1 Receptor Agonists	Albiglutide Dulaglutide Exenatide Liraglutide	Injection	No	Nausea Pancreatitis

Abbreviation: SGLT-2, sodium-glucose cotransporter-2.

WHEN TO START INSULIN?

The threshold glucose level that commands consideration of insulin is variable, depending on the resources of the patient and the expertise of the medical team. Historically, a glucose level greater than 200 mg/dL or an A1C level greater than 8% that is not responding to lifestyle and/or multiple oral medications is a concern that insulin may be necessary. Clearly, the presence of ketones in the urine and very high glucose level (ie, >300 mg/dL) is an indication for insulin therapy. The emergence of new classes of diabetes medications now allows the practitioner to try additional pills or injectable medications that can be started before using insulin. Many of these newer medications take weeks or months to reach full efficacy. If the patient has an urgent surgery date, it is advised to start insulin before the surgery date in order to reduce the risk for surgical complications. Commonly used insulins are listed in **Table 3**.

WHAT IS THE IMPACT OF POOR CONTROL ON SURGICAL OUTCOMES?

The diagnosis of diabetes increases the risk of perioperative complications. Postoperative hyperglycemia is associated with increased risk for complications in a continuous fashion above a threshold of 180 mg/dL.[8] For this reason, the ADA recommends that hospital glucose levels be maintained between 140 to 180 mg/dL.[9]

PARTNERING WITH A DIABETES SPECIALIST

The practice of medical diabetes management has grown in complexity. Medical therapy 20 years ago consisted of sulfonylureas, metformin, and insulin. New agents provide options and opportunities for better glycemic control, less weight gain, and reduced risk for cardiovascular events. The "down" side to these new therapies is that the patient must bear additional costs, because these new classes of medications are expensive. The practice of adding and adjusting multiple new diabetes medications is commonly beyond the scope of the busy primary practice physician. For this reason, the foot surgeon must confront the task of addressing the problem of poor glucose control in addition to providing expert podiatric and surgical care. In order to achieve good outcomes, limb salvage programs typically forge alliances with experts in diabetes care. Someone must take ownership of the diabetes care in order to achieve optimal surgical outcomes. This person may be the local diabetes center, an interested internist or family practitioner, or an endocrinologist. The ideal medical-surgical partnership provides the following:

Table 3
Commonly used insulins

Insulin Type	Onset of Action (Minutes)	Duration of Action (Hours)	Basal/Prandial Coverage
NPH	60	12–18	Basal
70/30	60	12–18	Both
Glargine	60	Up to 24	Basal
Detemir	60	Up to 24	Basal
Degludec	60–120	24–36	Basal
Regular	30	6–12	Prandial
Lispro	10–30	3–5	Prandial
Aspart	10–30	3–5	Prandial
Glulisine	10–30	3–5	Prandial

- Near same-day appointments for diabetes management
- DSMES
- Expert medical management, including initiating of insulin
- Timely communication to the limb salvage team and the primary care provider
- A return of the patient back to the primary care provider for routine care
- Timely communication to the foot surgeon and primary care provider on the status of the patient

PATIENT RESOURCES

The following nonprofit organizations provide a wealth of education and support to patients with diabetes. The organizations are supported by donations of time and money by persons with diabetes and their family members.

- ADA (www.diabetes.org)
- Joslin Diabetes Center (www.joslin.org)
- Taking Control of Your Diabetes (https://tcoyd.org)

SUMMARY

Both surgeons and clinicians must adjust to the growing epidemic of diabetes. The investment of time and energy for surgeons and clinicians to partner with each other will provide dividends in better surgical outcomes and healthier patients.

REFERENCES

1. Centers for Disease Control and Prevention, US Department of Health and Human Services. National diabetes statistics report 2017. 2017. Avialable at: https://www.cdc.gov/diabetes/data/statistics/statistics-report.html.
2. American Diabetes Association. Classification and diagnosis of diabetes: standards of medical care in diabetes-2018. Diabetes Care 2018;41(Suppl 1):S13–27.
3. American Diabetes Association. Glycemic targets: standards of medical care in diabetes-2018. Diabetes Care 2018;41(Suppl 1):S55–64.
4. Ortegon MM, Redekop WK, Niessen LW. Cost-effectiveness of prevention and treatment of the diabetic foot: a markov analysis. Diabetes Care 2004;27(4):901–7.
5. Davies MJ, D'Alessio DA, Fradkin J, et al. Management of hyperglycemia in type 2 diabetes, 2018. A consensus report by the american diabetes association (ADA) and the european association for the study of diabetes (EASD). Diabetes Care 2018;41(12):2669–701. Avialable at: https://www.ncbi.nlm.nih.gov/pubmed/30291106.
6. American diabetes association education recognition program. Avialable at: https://professional.diabetes.org/diabetes-education.
7. American Diabetes Association. Lifestyle management: standards of medical care in diabetes-2018. Diabetes Care 2018;41(Suppl 1):S38–50.
8. Frisch A, Chandra P, Smiley D, et al. Prevalence and clinical outcome of hyperglycemia in the perioperative period in noncardiac surgery. Diabetes Care 2010;33(8):1783–8.
9. American Diabetes Association. Diabetes care in the hospital: standards of medical care in diabetes-2018. Diabetes Care 2018;41(Suppl 1):S144–51.

Diabetic Foot Syndrome in the Twenty-First Century

Lawrence A. Lavery, DPM, MPH[a],*, Orhan K. Oz, MD, PhD[b], Kavitha Bhavan, MD[c], Dane K. Wukich, MD[d]

KEYWORDS

- Diabetes • Infection • Charcot • Arthropathy • Non-union • Ulcer • Neuropathy
- Amputation

KEY POINTS

- There are evolving innovative technologies, such as home temperature monitoring, negative pressure wound therapy, hyperspectral imaging, topical oxygen, and stem cell–based products, and a growing interest and investment by industry to improve the diagnosis and treatment of diabetic foot–related complications.
- The advances in vascular surgery, particularly endovascular interventions, also have contributed immensely to improved outcomes and reduced surgical risks.
- There has been the development and implementation of international treatment guidelines for the diabetic foot and growing implementation of diabetic foot programs from Tanzania to New York City.

INTRODUCTION

The first issue in Clinics in Podiatric Medicine dedicated to the diabetic foot was edited by Lawrence Harkless and Ken Dennis in 1987, over 30 years ago. The first diabetic foot issue had little evidence to advance the discussion or provide evidence to help direct therapy. Most of the papers were based on personal anecdotal experience. However, if you review the diabetic foot issue by Harkless and Dennis, there is a thread of truth that has contributed to the innovations and advances reported in the articles in this latest issue on the diabetic foot. The depth and quality of the

Disclose statement: Dr L.A. Lavery has a consulting agreement with eKare, EO2 Concepts, Bayer-Cardinal Health, KCI and he receives research funding from EO2 Concepts, Cardinal Health, KCI consulting, Avazzia, and Pluristem Therapeutics. The remaining authors have nothing to disclose.
[a] Department of Plastic Surgery, University of Texas Southwestern Medical Center, 5323 Harry Hines Boulevard, F4.310A, Dallas, TX 75390-8560, USA; [b] Department of Radiology, University of Texas Southwestern Medical Center, 5323 Harry Hines Boulevard, Dallas, TX 75390-8560, USA; [c] Department of Orthopaedic Surgery, University of Texas Southwestern Medical Center, 5323 Harry Hines Boulevard, Dallas, TX 75390-8560, USA; [d] Department of Internal Medicine, University of Texas Southwestern Medical Center, 5323 Harry Hines Boulevard, Dallas, TX 75390-8560, USA
* Corresponding author.
E-mail address: larry.lavery@utsouthwestern.edu

Clin Podiatr Med Surg 36 (2019) 355–359
https://doi.org/10.1016/j.cpm.2019.02.002
0891-8422/19/© 2019 Elsevier Inc. All rights reserved.

understanding of the diabetic foot disease process is apparent in the papers included in this text.

Diabetes is the epidemic of the twenty-first century. The prevalence of diabetes has exploded in the United States and around the world, and as would be expected, the incidence of diabetes-related complications has also demonstrated a dramatic increase. In developing countries 30 years ago, diabetes was uncommon, and today, China and India lead the world in the number of people with diabetes. And countries in the Middle East and Pacific Islands have the highest prevalence of diabetes.[1] In 2015, it was estimated that 415 million people globally had diabetes.[2] This is expected to increase to 642 million by 2040,[2] which represents a 55% increase in the next 2 decades. As a result of this epidemic, the global burden of diabetes and diabetic foot syndrome is expected to continue to increase.

The prevalence of diabetes and its related complications is growing in the United States, and the burden of diabetes is overwhelming the health care systems and disproportionately consuming health care resources. In 1990, the prevalence of diabetes in the United States was 2.5%, affecting 6.2 million people.[3] Over the past 30 years we have continually exceeded all projections regarding the prevalence of diabetes and the burden of diabetes-related complications. In just the 5-year period from 2007 to 2012, there was a 27% increase in the prevalence of diabetes in the United States,[4] increasing from 17.5 to 22.3 million patients. By 2017 there were 24.7 million people in the United States who were diagnosed with diabetes, afflicting 9.7% of the adult population.[5] This represents about a 4-fold increase in the number of Americans with diabetes since 1990.

The prevalence of diabetes increases with age, and it is disproportionately higher in minorities in the United States. In the US Medicare population, the prevalence of diabetes is estimated to be 25%. Native Americans, Pacific Islanders, African Americans, and people of Hispanic ancestry experience a higher prevalence of diabetes than Caucasians. Consequently, minority populations have a higher incidence of amputations, end-stage renal disease, and peripheral artery disease than Caucasians. For instance, the prevalence of diabetes in non-Hispanic white men and women in 2013 was 8.1/6.8%, compared with 12.6/11.7% in Hispanic Americans and 12.2/13.2% in African Americans.[6] Across all race and ethnic groups, men have a 2-fold higher incidence of amputation. After controlling for age, the incidence of amputation is 1.5 times higher in Hispanic Americans and 2 times higher in African Americans compared with Caucasians in the United States.[7]

The direct and indirect costs of diabetes result in a tremendous economic burden, and the increasing cost per patient is escalating at a higher rate than the increasing prevalence of diabetes. Diabetic patients on average have medical expenditures that are 2.3 times higher than patients without diabetes.[5] In 2017, the total estimated cost of patients diagnosed with diabetes was $327 billion, including $237 billion in direct medical costs and $90 billion in reduced productivity. The cost of diabetes increased by 41% from 2007 to 2012 and by an additional 25% from 2012 to 2017.[5,8]

Diabetic foot syndrome is a constellation of disease processes that are caused or exacerbated by diabetes. Similar to metastatic cancer, diabetes affects multiple organ systems and is associated with substantial morbidity and mortality. Unfortunately, patients do not view a diagnosis of diabetes in the same light as cancer despite its impact on multiple systems (cardiovascular, endocrine, immunologic, musculoskeletal, neurologic, ophthalmologic, renal). This translates into an exceptionally vulnerable population with very high prevalence and incidence rates of peripheral arterial disease (PAD), peripheral neuropathies, postural instability, osteopenia, osteoporosis, fractures, Charcot neuroarthropathy, ulcers, infections, and amputations. The prevalence of sensory neuropathy is 29% to 56% in adults with diabetes,[9–11] and the prevalence of PAD is 13.5% to 36%.[12] Approximately 592,000 patients with diabetes were living with a lower extremity amputation in 2005, and 60% of these were major amputations. The number of people living with an amputation is expected to increase by 70% by 2020,[13] and this cohort of patients is particularly vulnerable to further ulceration, infection, and amputation, often in the contralateral limb. Without preventive services and vigilant care, 50% to 80% of patients will have a new or recurrent ulcer in the next year. With standard prevention services, this high recurrent incidence can be cut in half.[14–16]

Diabetic foot ulcers (DFUs) are one of the pivotal factors that contribute to infection and limb loss.[17] Eight-five percent of diabetes-related amputations are preceded by an ulcer. To provide effective assessment, treatment of complications, and prevention services, it is imperative to understand the cause of DFUs. The cause of DFUs is usually multifactorial, developing in patients with peripheral sensory neuropathy, biomechanical abnormalities of the foot and ankle, external trauma, and macro- and microvascular disease. DFUs usually occur at the site of moderate or high foot pressure and shear forces that are exposed to repetitive trauma. Because of sensory neuropathy, patients often do not recognize the presence of a foot ulcer. Sites of abnormal pressure and shear are often associated with limited joint mobility and rigid structural foot deformities such as hammer toes, hallux valgus, hallux rigidus, equinus, and Charcot deformity.[17–19] Once a foot ulcer develops, the risk of infection increases dramatically, and up to 60% of patients will develop infection. Approximately 80% of infections are soft tissue, whereas 20% are bone infections.[11,20] Patients with diabetes have about a 4- to 9.5-fold increased risk of infection compared with people without diabetes.[21,22] There are several factors that may explain the high rate of infection. Patients with diabetes and neuropathy present later for care than people without diabetes with infection[23,24] due to sensory neuropathy and minimal pain. Diabetic patients have deficits in humoral and cellular immunity that may impair the normal host response to bacterial infection.[25–27] Finally, patients with diabetes have macro- and micro-peripheral vascular disease that may impair tissue penetration with antibiotics and impede healing.

The role of the multidisciplinary team to treat and prevent diabetic foot complications has been the corner stone of treatment and the inspiration for scientific meetings for the past 30 years.[28] There are 19 studies that report the impact of a team approach to diabetic limb salvage. Although the specific team members vary from site to site, diabetic foot care providers are often driven by their interest in the topic rather than by their degree or specialty. The outcomes that are reported are quite variable as well, but reduction in the incidence of amputations, reduction in high-level amputations, improved wound healing, reduced length of stay, and reduced reulceration are common outcomes associated with a multidisciplinary team. Diabetic foot teams should strive for the same success seen in centers that specialize in trauma, heart attack, and stroke. The improved outcomes seen in patients with trauma, heart attack, and stroke are due to the following: (1) a team-based approach to care, (2) evidence-based protocols, (3) commitment from hospital leadership, and (4) providers with expertise who are passionately dedicated to measuring quality and improving patient care.

The understanding of diabetic foot syndrome has dramatically improved over the past decades. There has been the development and implementation of international treatment guidelines for the diabetic foot and growing implementation of diabetic foot programs from Tanzania to New York City. There is a growing body of high-quality, multidisciplinary peer reviewed literature that has expanded the authors' knowledge and challenged their clinical practices. There are evolving innovative technologies, such as home temperature monitoring, negative pressure wound therapy, hyperspectral imaging, topical oxygen, and stem cell–based products, and a growing interest and investment by industry to improve the diagnosis and treatment of diabetic foot–related complications. The advances in vascular surgery, particularly endovascular interventions, also have contributed immensely to improved outcomes and reduced surgical risks. There are new procedures and approaches to reconstruct Charcot neuroarthropathy and improve sensory neuropathy that were not considered 30 years ago. Although the treatment protocols and outcomes have advanced significantly over the past several decades, much remains to be done. This is an exciting time for those who treat diabetes-related foot complications. The authors hope that this issue will inspire the next generation of clinicians and researchers to continue to advance the understanding and clinical practice of the diabetic foot syndrome. The German philosopher Arthur Schopenhauer (1788–1860) stated that "a talented person hits a target no one else can hit. A genius hits a target that no one else can see." Maybe one of the readers will be that genius.

REFERENCES

1. Naeem Z. Burden of diabetes mellitus in Saudi Arabia. Int J Health Sci (Qassim) 2015;9(3). V–VI.
2. Ogurtsova K, da Rocha Fernandes JD, Huang Y, et al. IDF Diabetes Atlas: global estimates for the prevalence of diabetes for 2015 and 2040. Diabetes Res Clin Pract 2017;128:40–50.
3. CDC's Division of Diabetes Translation. Long-term Trends in Diabetes. United States Diabetes Surveillance System; 2017. Available at: http://www.cdc.gov/diabetes/data.
4. American Diabetes Association. Economic costs of diabetes in the U.S. in 2012. Diabetes Care 2013;36(4):1033–46.
5. American Diabetes Association. Economic costs of diabetes in the U.S. In 2017. Diabetes Care 2018;41(5):917–28.
6. CDC. Estimates of diabetes and its burden in the United States. National diabetes statistics report, 2017. Atlanta (GA): CDC; 2017.
7. Lefebvre KM, Lavery LA. Disparities in amputations in minorities. Clin Orthop Relat Res 2011;469(7):1941–50.
8. Reiber GE, Vileikyte L, Boyko EJ, et al. Causal pathways for incident lower-extremity ulcers in patients with diabetes from two settings. Diabetes Care 1999;22(1):157–62.
9. Bansal D, Gudala K, Muthyala H, et al. Prevalence and risk factors of development of peripheral diabetic neuropathy in type 2 diabetes mellitus in a tertiary care setting. J Diabetes Investig 2014;5(6):714–21.
10. Lazo Mde L, Bernabe-Ortiz A, Pinto ME, et al. Diabetic peripheral neuropathy in ambulatory patients with type 2 diabetes in a general hospital in a middle income country: a cross-sectional study. PLoS One 2014;9(5):e95403.
11. Lavery LA, Armstrong DG, Wunderlich RP, et al. Diabetic foot syndrome: evaluating the prevalence and incidence of foot pathology in Mexican Americans and non-Hispanic whites from a diabetes disease management cohort. Diabetes Care 2003;26(5):1435–8.
12. Shukla V, Fatima J, Ali M, et al. A study of prevalence of peripheral arterial disease in type 2 diabetes mellitus patients in a Teaching Hospital. J Assoc Physicians India 2018;66(5):57–60.
13. Ziegler-Graham K, MacKenzie EJ, Ephraim PL, et al. Estimating the prevalence of limb loss in the United States: 2005 to 2050. Arch Phys Med Rehabil 2008;89(3):422–9.

14. Lavery LA, La Fontaine J, Kim PJ. Preventing the first or recurrent ulcers. Med Clin North Am 2013;97(5):807–20.
15. Lavery LA, Peters EJ, Williams JR, et al, International Working Group on the Diabetic Foot. Reevaluating the way we classify the diabetic foot: restructuring the diabetic foot risk classification system of the International Working Group on the Diabetic Foot. Diabetes Care 2008;31(1):154–6.
16. Peters EJ, Lavery LA, International Working Group on the Diabetic F. Effectiveness of the diabetic foot risk classification system of the International Working Group on the Diabetic Foot. Diabetes Care 2001;24(8):1442–7.
17. Lavery LA, Peters EJ, Armstrong DG. What are the most effective interventions in preventing diabetic foot ulcers? Int Wound J 2008;5(3):425–33.
18. Peters EJ, Armstrong DG, Lavery LA. Risk factors for recurrent diabetic foot ulcers: site matters. Diabetes Care 2007;30(8):2077–9.
19. Lavery LA, Armstrong DG, Boulton AJ, et al. Ankle equinus deformity and its relationship to high plantar pressure in a large population with diabetes mellitus. J Am Podiatr Med Assoc 2002;92(9):479–82.
20. Lavery LA, Armstrong DG, Wunderlich RP, et al. Risk factors for foot infections in individuals with diabetes. Diabetes Care 2006;29(6):1288–93.
21. Wukich DK, McMillen RL, Lowery NJ, et al. Surgical site infections after foot and ankle surgery: a comparison of patients with and without diabetes. Diabetes Care 2011;34(10):2211–3.
22. Wukich DK, Lowery NJ, McMillen RL, et al. Postoperative infection rates in foot and ankle surgery: a comparison of patients with and without diabetes mellitus. J Bone Joint Surg Am 2010;92(2):287–95.
23. Armstrong DG, Lavery LA, Quebedeaux TL, et al. Surgical morbidity and the risk of amputation due to infected puncture wounds in diabetic versus nondiabetic adults. South Med J 1997;90(4):384–9.
24. Lavery LA, Walker SC, Harkless LB, et al. Infected puncture wounds in diabetic and nondiabetic adults. Diabetes Care 1995;18(12):1588–91.
25. Wada J, Makino H. Innate immunity in diabetes and diabetic nephropathy. Nat Rev Nephrol 2016;12(1):13–26.
26. Zhou T, Hu Z, Yang S, et al. Role of adaptive and innate immunity in type 2 diabetes mellitus. J Diabetes Res 2018;2018:7457269.
27. Joseph WS, LeFrock JL. The pathogenesis of diabetic foot infections–immunopathy, angiopathy, and neuropathy. J Foot Surg 1987;26(1 Suppl):S7–11.
28. Buggy A, Moore Z. The impact of the multidisciplinary team in the management of individuals with diabetic foot ulcers: a systematic review. J Wound Care 2017; 26(6):324–39.

Perfusion Assessment and Treatment in the Diabetic Patient

Michael Cyrus Siah, MD, Steven Abramowitz, MD*

KEYWORDS

- Perfusion • Angiography • Endovascular • Surgical bypass
- Noninvasive vascular studies

KEY POINTS

- Pulse examination and the ankle-brachial index are critical ways to assess blood flow in the lower extremity at the bedside.
- A clinician's assessment can be augmented with the use of noninvasive arterial studies such as toe systolic pressure measurements, transcutaneous partial oxygen pressure measurements, pulse volume recordings, and hyperspectral imaging.
- Noninvasive diagnostic imaging using duplex ultrasonography, computed tomography, and magnetic resonance angiography provides critical preoperative planning information prior to revascularization.
- The decision between endovascular and open therapeutic interventions is nuanced and related to a variety of factors including patient comorbidities, lesion length and characteristics, and the presence of autogenous conduit.

INTRODUCTION

Many studies have established the association between diabetes mellitus and peripheral arterial disease (PAD). Although atherosclerosis is a generalized process that can occur in diabetics and nondiabetics alike, the prevalence of PAD is more common in diabetic patients. In patients with diabetes, for every 1% increase in hemoglobin A1c, there is a 26% associated increase in the risk of PAD.[1] In fact, PAD in conjunction with diabetic neuropathy, contributes to 50% of diabetic foot ulcerations.[2]

The predominant arterial beds impacted by PAD in the diabetic patient are typically infrageniculate, or below the knee. The pathophysiologic mechanism of disease of the anterior tibial, posterior tibial, peroneal, dorsalis pedis, and geniculate arteries is most

---

Disclosure Statement: The authors have nothing to disclose.
Department of Vascular Surgery, MedStar Washington Hospital Center, 106 Irving Street Northwest POB North 3150, Washington, DC 20010, USA
* Corresponding author.
E-mail address: steven.abramowitz@medstar.net

Clin Podiatr Med Surg 36 (2019) 361–370
https://doi.org/10.1016/j.cpm.2019.03.001
0891-8422/19/© 2019 Elsevier Inc. All rights reserved.

frequently medial calcinosis.[3] Below the ankle, the inframalleolar and pedal arch vessels may be impacted by nonenzymatic glycation caused by elevated blood sugar.[4] Disease in any vascular bed may impact wound healing. For example, even an incomplete pedal arch is associated with recurrent ulceration within 1 year after primary ulcer healing.[5] These implications highlight the importance of vigilant perfusion screening in both symptomatic and asymptomatic diabetic patients to improve the healing of and prevent new and recurrent ulcerations.

PHYSICAL EXAMINATION

Perfusion assessment of the diabetic patient begins with a well-documented physical assessment prior to pulse examination. It should include gross examination of the patient for the stigmata of peripheral vascular disease. Examination of each limb should identify scars indicating healed arterial or venous ulcers and prior surgical interventions such as saphenous vein harvesting or distal bypass and biomechanical callous formation. Trophic skin lesions such as pale, cool skin or shiny, thickened nail beds, may be visible. Hair loss is an unreliable sign of ischemia and is of little clinical value.[6] Capillary refill in the soft tissue or under the nail bed should be assessed. Atrophy, pallor, and asymmetric peripheral temperatures should be noted. Ulcerations and areas of necrosis or gangrene should be described, measured, and photographed.

The pulse examination is the most critical component of the physical examination. Identification of diminished or absent pedal pulses provides a general indication as to the presence and level of atherosclerotic disease burden. For example, a palpable popliteal pulse in the setting of absent pedal pulses suggests isolated tibial disease, whereas an absent popliteal pulse may suggest a more proximal disease burden. Regardless of the level of disease, the UK National Institute for Health and Care Excellence (NICE) National Guidelines for the diabetic foot suggest that the absence of palpable pedal pulses is sufficient for the identification of vascular impairment.[7] Any atherosclerotic disease resulting in the loss of a pulse may cause inadequate perfusion for wound healing.[3]

There are many published scales that may aid in the standardization of physical examination reporting. Consistent use allows for the clinician to track patient improvement or decline. The Fontaine and Rutherford classifications and the University of Texas system have historically been used to guide wound assessments; however, each do not incorporate all of the etiologies of threatened limbs. The presence of infection and involvement of deeper structures increase the metabolic requirement of ulcer healing.[8] To account for this, the Society for Vascular Surgery devised the Wound Ischemia and Foot Infection (WIfI) System to better predict amputation risk and better evaluate outcomes in the treatment of peripheral vascular disease. By integrating the key factors associated with tissue loss, the WIfI classification system is able to combine perfusion and tissue assessment to better predict clinical outcomes than previous scoring systems. Ultimately, the use of any of these scoring systems allows for objective assessment of patients that can guide care and monitor outcomes.

NONINVASIVE PERFUSION ASSESSMENT

Noninvasive testing is beneficial in both the diagnosis of existing peripheral vascular disease and in screening patients for advancing atherosclerotic disease. The simplest of noninvasive examination that can be performed is the ankle-brachial index (ABI). It is a critical extension of the vascular physical examination and can be performed by the clinician at the bedside. The ABI is a ratio of the ankle and brachial systolic blood pressures. A normal ABI can range from 0.9 to 1.2.[9] Generally, an ABI of greater than 0.8 is not associated with impaired wound healing.[10] Given the ease with which an ABI can be performed, the American Diabetes Association recommends PAD screening with an ABI every 5 years in patients with diabetes.[11]

Unfortunately, ABI values can often be unreliable in the diabetic patient because of the extensive calcification, or medial calcinosis, of the infrapopliteal blood vessels. This extensive calcification prevents proper compression of the tibial arteries and results in either a falsely elevated ABI or a value that is unattainable because of the inability to achieve vessel compression at a suprasystolic cuff pressure. Therefore, any abnormal, be it diminished or falsely elevated (noncompressible), ABI indicates the presence of arterial disease that should be further evaluated.

When ABIs are impaired or unattainable, a vascular laboratory can provide other useful diagnostic tests to assess perfusion in the diabetic patient. Pulse volume recording (PVR), also known as plethysmography, is a noninvasive method to evaluate the arteries of the lower extremity. Segmental pressures and waveforms are analyzed to identify the level and degree of potential stenosis. Pressure cuffs are used to measure the pulsatile change in blood pressure at various levels of a limb. Abnormal PVR findings include decreased amplitude, a flattened peak, and an absent dicrotic notch. Amplitudes of less than 5 mm from trough to peak have been used as a criterion for the diagnosis of peripheral vascular disease[12] (**Fig. 1**).

Toe systolic pressure measurement (TSP) and transcutaneous partial oxygen pressure measurement ($TcPO_2$) are useful modalities to attain a better understanding of tissue perfusion. The measurement of toe pressures allows for an accurate assessment of pedal perfusion, as digital vessels are often free of atherosclerotic disease burden. Toe pressures are usually 30 mm Hg less than ankle pressures, and an abnormal toe-brachial index (TBI) is <0.70.[13] However, digital ulceration or prior amputation may limit the usefulness of the TBI examination.

$TcPO_2$ of the partial oxygen pressure is performed at the back of the foot and between the first and second toe space. Normal $TcPO_2$ for a diabetic patient is 50 mm Hg.[14] Hafner[15] and Suzuki and colleagues[16] demonstrated pressures less than 30 mm Hg to be associated with severe ischemia, while pressures greater than 40 mm Hg are associated with wound healing with conservative therapy. Additionally, Kalani and colleagues[17] demonstrated that TcPO2 can be a better predictor for ulcer healing than toe pressures in diabetics with foot ulcerations and confirmed a low likelihood of wound healing with pressures less than 25 mm Hg. Therefore, the likelihood of wound healing increases with skin perfusion pressures of greater than 40 mm Hg, toe pressures greater than 30 mm Hg, or TcPO2 greater than 25 mm Hg.[18] Values below these levels suggest a role for invasive diagnostic and therapeutic measures. It should be noted, however, that despite the documented utility of skin perfusion pressure measurements and $TcPO_2$, they are not typically performed. $TcPO_2$ measurements may be influenced by many technical features, including the type of equipment used, monitor placement, and surface temperature of the measured area.

Hyperspectral imaging (HSI) has emerged as an additional noninvasive way to assess tissue perfusion and may have a role in predicting wound healing in diabetic patients with tissue loss. HSI identifies tissue oxygenation on a microvascular level and anatomically demonstrates changes in the microcirculation. Unlike TpCO2, HSI measurements can be performed quickly in the clinic. Additionally, HSI can directly evaluate perfusion in the ulcer bed. One of the major barriers to widespread application of the technology is cost, as the devices are generally expensive. Additionally,

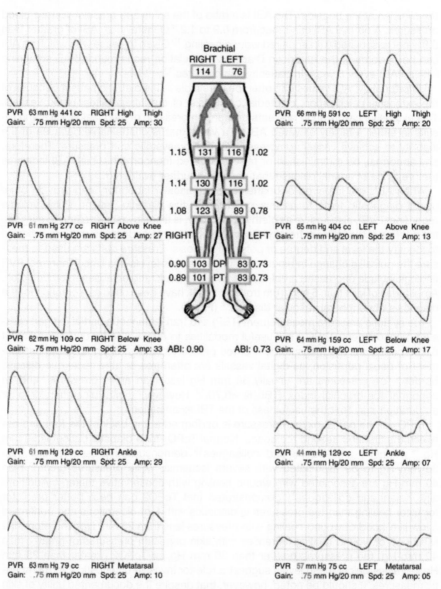

Fig. 1. Physiologic study demonstrating segmental pulse volume recording. (*From* Vascular Laboratory Testing. Vascular medicine: a companion to Braunwald's heart disease, by Creager MA, et al. Elsevier/Saunders, 2013, pp. 148–165; with permission)

there is a lack of evidence demonstrating the reliability of HIS measurements in diabetics with tissue loss (**Fig. 2**).

NONINVASIVE DIAGNOSTIC IMAGING

Of the many modalities available to assess the arterial supply of the lower extremity, the most commonly utilized are duplex ultrasound, computed tomography

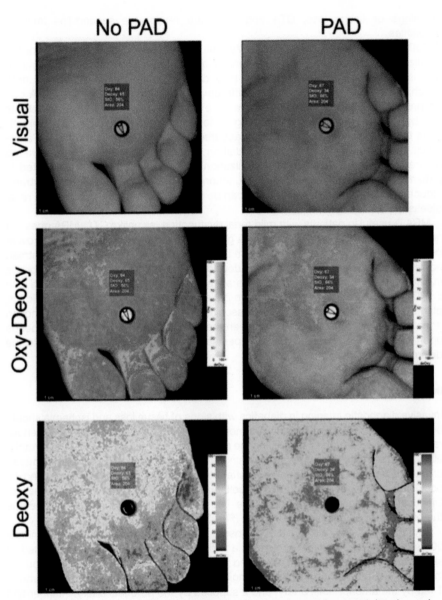

Fig. 2. Visual hyperspectral images of pedal perfusion in a foot with no peripheral vascular disease (*left*) and a foot with peripheral vascular disease (*right*). (*From* Chin JA, et al. Evaluation of hyperspectral technology for assessing the presence and severity of peripheral artery disease. Journal of Vascular Surgery 2011:54(6): 1679–1688. https://doi.org/10.1016/j.jvs. 2011.06.022; with permission.)

angiography (CTA), and magnetic resonance angiography (MRA). In general, these imaging tests should be reserved for patients prior to or after endovascular or surgical therapy. Ultrasound is considered to be the first-line study given its low cost and the lack of potentially adverse side effects. In patients in whom ultrasound is unlikely to be successful, particularly patients who have morbid obesity or extensive dressings or tissue loss, CTA and MRA are reasonable second-line imaging modalities.

Both CTA and MRA allow for visualization of suprainguinal blood vessels, for the localization of infrainguinal disease burden, and the characterization of stenotic or occlusive lesions. Most importantly, they can show the quality of tibial runoff, which is vital for deciding between different interventional strategies. A CTA can be performed rapidly and allows for easy evaluation of previously placed stents and bypasses. However, in the setting of severe calcification, CTA may overestimate the degree of stenosis and lack accuracy of flow assessment of the tibial arteries. Additionally, CTA requires radiation exposure and the use of iodinated contrast agents for vasculature visualization. Such agents are contraindicated in patients with underlying renal dysfunction because of the risk of contrast-induced nephropathy. However, they can be used in patients with end -stage renal disease (ESRD).

MRA is useful in patients with mild renal dysfunction, as unlike CTA, MRA does not require iodinated contrast. MRA uses a gadolinium-based contrast agent to provide better visualization of the arterial system in the lower extremity. Gadolinium contrast, however, has been associated with the development of nephrogenic systemic fibrosis in patients with impaired creatinine clearance and is contraindicated in patients with ESRD. MRA utilization may be limited in patients with claustrophobia or metallic implants, and long acquisition times are associated with more patient-generated motion artifact. Ultimately, the selection between the use of duplex, CTA, or MRA depends upon patient specific factors, local expertise, and safety profile and are up to the discretion of the clinician.

INVASIVE DIAGNOSTIC IMAGING

Invasive diagnostic imaging in diabetics with signs of tissue loss and ischemia should be limited to those patients who would not benefit from primary amputation. Arteriography is the best means of identifying the distribution and extent of PAD. Angiography allows for real-time flow assessment using either carbon dioxide, iodinated contrast, or gadolinium contrast to visualize arterial flow under fluoroscopy. Arterial stenosis, occlusive lesions, and named vessel collateral reconstitution may all be assessed. Diagnostic imaging may then translate into endovascular intervention or become the basis for open surgical intervention (**Fig. 3**).

Angiography also allows for angiosome characterization. Introduced nearly 30 years ago, an angiosome refers to a 3-dimensional unit of tissue comprised of skin, subcutaneous tissue, muscle, and bone, supplied by a clear arterial source. In the lower leg and foot, there are 6 angiosomes: 3 fed by the posterior tibial artery, 1 fed by the anterior tibial artery, and 2 supplied by the peroneal artery. Attinger and colleagues[19] have demonstrated the validity of the angiosome concept in free flap procedures; however, the data regarding the angiosome in diabetic patients with PAD are less conclusive.

The clinical application of the angiosome concept requires an understanding of perfusion sources of the foot and considering these as therapeutic targets for intervention. Interventionalists can perform angiosome-directed revascularization procedures, which focus on intervening on the source vessel/angiosome of ulceration, as opposed to indirect revascularization procedures. Some studies have demonstrated more rapid times to healing with angiosome-directed revascularization procedures, however no difference in amputation rates. Ultimately, considering the option of angiosome–directed revascularization should be performed;

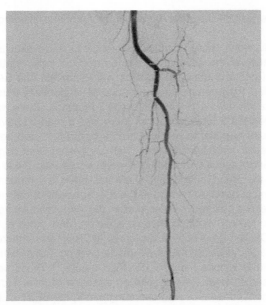

Fig. 3. Diagnostic arteriogram revealing flush occlusion of the anterior tibial artery and a long segment posterior tibial artery occlusion. (*From* Tsubakimoto Y. TCTAP C-201 successful limb salvage in a CLI patient with scleroderma by complete revascularization of BTA lesions. Journal of the American College of Cardiology 2015;65(17) . https://doi.org/10.1016/j.jacc. 2015.03.485; with permission.)

however, revascularization should still be pursued indirectly if no direct revascularization targets are available.

Given the challenge of correlating angiosomes- and nonangiosomes-based perfusion assessment with clinical outcomes, the use of indocyanine green angiography (ICGA) has also emerged as perfusion assessment tool. ICGA has been studied extensively in free flap creation and has been shown to provide perfusion information that predicts tissue survival in assessing flap viability.[20–22] ICG is administered intravascularly and binds to serum proteins. The uptake of ICG can be quantified in the tissue bed of interest, and this value may serve as a surrogate for tissue perfusion. Ongoing studies are being performed to determine the role of IGCA for optimal treatment of peripheral vascular disease, as well as to assess the success of revascularization procedures.[23,24]

THERAPEUTIC OPTIONS

There are 2 modalities to address perfusion deficits in diabetic patients with tissue loss: open and endovascular surgery. Open techniques, namely surgical bypass, historically have been the mainstay of treatment. Bypass with autogenous conduit, most commonly the greater saphenous vein, represents the gold standard for revascularization techniques, as it is associated with better patency and increased amputation-free survival compared with bypass using prosthetic conduits.[25] However, endovascular therapies have emerged as an acceptable first-line treatment in the surgical management of ischemic diabetic foot ulcerations. This is likely because of the ease with which diagnostic and therapeutic procedures can now be performed, as well as the wide variety of interventionalists who are capable of performing them.

Coming to a decision between bypass first versus an endovascular first strategy is challenging because of the absence of randomized controlled data demonstrating the superiority of either modality in patients with diabetes. The BASIL trial, a randomized controlled trial, compared the results of angioplasty versus bypass and examined amputation rates and survival for the 2 methods. There was no significant difference between the 2 techniques, but there was a marked advantage of endovascular techniques in patients with elevated surgical risk, and better results than prosthetic bypasses. Additionally, the trial suggested that bypass outcomes following failed endovascular interventions were worse than those performed prior to endovascular therapy. Since BASIL, there has been few randomized controlled data to guide clinical decision making in the management of critical limb ischemia, but there has been a marked proliferation in the endovascular tools available to interventionalists. Newer wires, catheters, sheaths, and other devices like drug-eluting stents (DESs), drug-coated balloons (DCBs), and atherectomy devices have become readily available and have made treating TransAtlantic Inter-Society Consensus C and D lesions much easier than before.[18] These newer techniques are frequently used to treat PAD despite an absence of level 1 data. To address the lack of treatment consensus in PAD management, the BEST-CLI (Best Endovascular vs Best Surgical Therapy for Patients With Critical Limb Ischemia) trial is being conducted. This trial will compare outcomes of the best endovascular and open surgical revascularization strategies in patients with tissue loss and infrainguinal PAD.

SUMMARY

PAD in the diabetic patient is a growing problem and will continue to represent a tremendous economic and social burden facing modern societies in the 21st century. Early recognition of perfusion deficits is critical in curtailing the extent of this problem, and there are several noninvasive tests that allow for the objective identification of PAD. Once diagnosed, referral to a vascular specialist allows for restoration of arterial perfusion, either by open or endovascular techniques.

REFERENCES

1. Selvin E, Marinopoulos S, Berkenblit G, et al. Meta-analysis: glycosylated hemoglobin and cardiovascular disease in diabetes mellitus. Ann Intern Med 2004; 141(6):421–31. www.ncbi.nlm.nih.gov/pubmed/15381515.
2. Prompers L, Schaper N, Apelqvist J, et al. Prediction of outcome in individuals with diabetic footulcers: focus on the differences between individuals with and without peripheral arterial disease. The EURODIALE Study. Diabetologia 2008; 51:747–55.
3. Ho CY, Shanahan CM. Medial arterial calcification: an overlooked player in peripheral arterial disease. Arterioscler Thromb Vasc Biol 2016. https://doi.org/10.1161/ATVBAHA.116.306717.
4. Schalkwijk CG, Miyata T. Early- and advanced non-enzymatic glycation in diabetic vascular complications: the search for therapeutics. Amino Acids 2010; 42(4):1193–204.
5. Pound N, Chipchase S, Treece K, et al. Ulcer-free survival following management of foot ulcers in diabetes. Diabet Med 2005;22:1306–9.

6. Golomb BA, Dang TT, Criqui MH. Peripheral arterial disease: morbidity and mortality implications. Circulation 2006;114:688–99.

7. Bailey MA, Griffin KJ, Scott DJ. Clinical assessment of patients with peripheral arterial disease. Semin Intervent Radiol 2014;31(4):292–9.

8. Diabetic foot problems: prevention and management. Guidance and Guidelines | NICE. Available at: www.nice.org.uk/guidance/ng19. Accessed December 22, 2018.

9. Weitz JI, Byrne J, Clagett GP, et al. Diagnosis and treatment of chronic arterial insufficiency of the lower extremities: a critical review. Circulation 1996;94(11): 3026–49.

10. Mills JL. Lower limb ischaemia in patients with diabetic foot ulcers and gangrene: recognition, anatomic patterns and revascularization strategies. Diabetes Metab Res Rev 2016;32:239–45.

11. American Diabetes Association. Peripheral arterial disease in people with diabetes. Diabetes Care 2003;26(12):3333–41.

12. Sacks D. The TransAtlantic Inter-Society consensus (TASC) on the management of peripheral arterial disease. J Vasc Interv Radiol 2003;14(9). https://doi.org/10.1097/01.rvi.0000094603.61428.1c.

13. Vayssairat M. VII. Microcirculatory explorations. J Mal Vasc 2002;27:2803.

14. Sibley RC, Reis SP, MacFarlane JJ, et al. Noninvasive physiologic vascular studies: a guide to diagnosing peripheral arterial disease. Radiographics 2017; 37(1):346–57.

15. Hafner J. Management of arterial leg ulcers and of combined (mixed) venous-arterial leg ulcers. Curr Probl Dermatol 1999;27:211–9.

16. Suzuki K, Birnbaum Z, Lockhart R, et al. Skin perfusion pressure and wound closure time in lower extremity wounds. J Am Coll Clin Wound Spec 2017; 9(1–3):14–8.

17. Kalani M, Brismar K, Fagrell B, et al. Transcutaneous oxygen tension and toe blood pressure as predictors for outcome of diabetic foot ulcers. Diabetes Care 1999;22(1):147–51.

18. Goodney PP, Beck A, Welch HG, et al. National trends in lower extremity bypass surgery, endovascular interventions and major amputations. J Vasc Surg 2009; 50(1):54–60..

19. Attinger CE, Evans KK, Bulan E, et al. Angiosomes of the foot and ankle and clinical implications for limb salvage: reconstruction, incisions, and revascularization. Plast Reconstr Surg 2006;117(7 Supplement):261S–93S.

20. Newman MI, Samson MC, Tamburrino JF, et al. Intra- operative laser-assisted indocyanine green angiography for the evaluation of mastectomy flaps in immediate breast recon- struction. J Reconstr Microsurg 2010;26:487–92.

21. Pestana I, Coan B, Erdmann D, et al. Early experience with fluorescent angiography in free-tissue transfer reconstruction. Plast Reconstr Surg 2009;123: 1239–44.

22. Igari K, Kudo T, Uchiyama H, et al. Indocyanine green angiography for the diagnosis of peripheral arterial disease with isolated infrapopliteal lesions. Ann Vasc Surg 2014;28(6):1479–84.

23. Igari K, Kudo T, Toyofuku T, et al. Quantitative evaluation of the outcomes of revascularization procedures for peripheral arterial disease using indocyanine green angiography. Eur J Vasc Endovasc Surg 2013;46(4):460–5.

24. Brownrigg JRW, Hinchliffe RJ, Apelqvist J, et al. Performance of prognostic markers in the prediction of wound healing or amputation among patients with

foot ulcers in diabetes: a systematic review. Diabetes Metab Res Rev 2016;32: 128–35.

25. Adam DJ, Beard JD, Cleveland T, et al. Bypass versus angioplasty in severe ischaemia of the leg (BASIL): multicentre, randomised controlled trial. Lancet 2005;366(9501):1925–34.

Conservative Offloading

Peter A. Crisologo, DPM[a], Lawrence A. Lavery, DPM, MPH[b],
Javier La Fontaine, DPM, MS[b],*

KEYWORDS

- Diabetes • Offloading • Ulcer • Deformity

KEY POINTS

- Diabetic ulcers develop in areas of pressure.
- Neuropathy is essential for development of this ulcer. Deformities need to be recognized and accommodated with offloading devices.
- Global factors, including blindness, limited joint mobility, and obesity often are obstacles for proper offloading.
- Total contact cast is the gold standard for offloading a neuropathic ulcer.

INTRODUCTION

The etiology of ulcerations in diabetes mellitus is associated with the presence of peripheral sensory neuropathy and repetitive trauma due to normal walking activities to areas on the foot that are subject to moderate or high pressures and shear.[1] Pressure sites on the sole of the foot are often associated with limited joint mobility of the foot or ankle or structure deformities such as hammertoes and hallux valgus deformity. The combination of loss of protective sensation, deformity, and repetitive trauma is the perfect storm for ulcer development. Once an ulcer is developed, the most important part of the healing process is offloading the ulcer site. Unfortunately, other comorbid factors such as blindness, loss of proprioception, prior amputations, and obesity make non–weight-bearing status impossible. The goal of this article is to provide the reader with the best evidence supported options for offloading of the diabetic foot ulceration, that could be applied to their patient population.

EVALUATING FOOT DEFORMITY IN PATIENTS WITH DIABETES

In patients with neuropathy, ulcerations typically develop as a result of repetitive pressure and shear on the sole of the foot or from shoe pressure on the top or sides of the

Disclosure Statement: The authors have nothing to disclose.
[a] Department of Plastic Surgery, UT Southwestern Medical Center, 5323 Harry Hines Boulevard, Dallas, TX 75390, USA; [b] Department of Plastic Surgery and Orthopaedic Surgery, UT Southwestern Medical Center, 5323 Harry Hines Boulevard, Dallas, TX 75390, USA
* Corresponding author.
E-mail address: javier.lafontaine@utsouthwestern.edu

foot; however, no specific level of pressure has been determined to be abnormal or pathologic.[2] Diabetes alters biomechanics in patients with preexisting structural and functional foot deformities. Motor neuropathy is thought to contribute to atrophy and weakness of the intrinsic muscles of the foot. This leads to what has been called the "intrinsic minus foot," which describes wasting of the small (intrinsic) muscles that originate in the foot (see **Fig. 4**).

Metatarsal ulcers can develop when digital deformities severely contract. The lesser digits contract and dislocate dorsally, resulting in a claw toe deformity and a strong plantar flexor force at the metatarsophalangeal joints. As the toes contract and the metatarsophalangeal joints dislocate, retrograde forces push the metatarsal heads plantarly.[3] Therefore, 3 areas are subject to excessive pressure: the distal tip of the toes, dorsal aspect of the lesser digits, and the metatarsal heads, which in the presence of loss of protective sensation, can lead to ulceration.[4] Limited mobility of the ankle and metatarsophalangeal joints has been associated with soft tissue glycosylation involving the gastro-soleus-Achilles complex and periarticular tissues.[5] Limited motion of the ankle, subtalar, and metatarsophalangeal joints have been associated with high pressures in the forefoot. Often patients with an intrinsic minus foot will appear to have a high arch; however, this is not a congenital deformity but rather is due to atrophy of the abductor hallucis muscle belly on the medial side of the foot. A profound example of musculoskeletal abnormality of the diabetic foot is represented by Charcot neuroarthropathy, which is characterized by fracture, subluxation, and/or dislocation of joints in the foot or ankle. These structural deformities typically cause plantar bony deformities resulting in areas of high pressure leading to ulceration.

Reduction of pressure and shear forces on the foot may be the single most important yet most often neglected aspect of neuropathic ulcer treatment. Offloading therapy is a key part of the treatment plan for diabetic foot ulcers. The goal is to reduce the pressure at the ulcer site and keep the patient ambulatory.[6,7] Several methods are available to protect the foot from abnormal pressure. Offloading strategies must be tailored to the age, strength, activity, and home environment of the patient. In general, however, more restrictive offloading approaches will result in less activity and better wound healing. Education is critical to improve compliance with offloading. The patient must understand that the wound is a result of repetitive pressure and that every unprotected step is literally tearing the wound apart.

Offloading Shoes and Sandals

A number of offloading shoes and sandals or wedged offloading shoes are available to reduce pressure on the forefoot. These shoes are useful for patients who are not able to tolerate a total contact cast (TCC), other more appropriate methods of offloading, or for those who need a transitional device after removal of a TCC while they are awaiting custom-made therapeutic shoes and insoles.

Surgical shoes with a rocker sole design are preferable to the flat design (**Fig. 1**) for postoperative use. Some models of sandal use an insole with hex-shaped portions that can be removed to offload the ulceration, described previously, and can be used as a transitional device after closing the wound. The wedged shoe (**Fig. 2**) was originally designed to protect the forefoot after elective surgery. This shoe has a built-in 10-degree dorsiflexory angle, effectively removing pressure from the forefoot area and redistributing it to the hindfoot. However, these types of shoes are not tolerated well by patients because they are difficult to ambulate with. They typically cause pain of the contralateral extremity, and are often not safe for use in patients with gait and postural instability. Also, many people with diabetes have equinus and cannot tolerate the negative heel position created by the shoe. This dorsiflexory

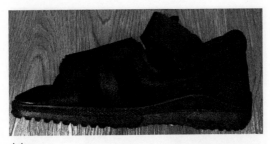

Fig. 1. Healing sandal.

angle causes suspension of the heel during ambulation and subsequently increases pressure on the forefoot and stresses the midfoot, a common site for collapse in the diabetic Charcot foot. In a randomized clinical trial that compared TCCs with healing sandals and removable cast boots, patients in the healing sandal group were less compliant and used the device during walking significantly less than did subjects in the TCC group.[8]

Ankle-Foot Custom-Made Orthoses

Custom-made ankle-foot orthoses are commonly used for moderate to severe lower-extremity. The Charcot Restraint Orthotic Walker (CROW) (**Fig. 3**), for example, was initially used to treat patients with neuropathic fractures, and who acquire rocker-bottom deformity. It provides protection to the neuropathic foot and aids in controlling lower-extremity edema. It also allows removal for dressing changes, but is also very rigid, preventing excessive motion. The rigid polypropylene shell with a rocker-bottom sole allows accommodation for severe deformities. The CROW can be adjusted and repaired when deformities change.

The primary drawback to custom-made devices is that they are very expensive and a good technician is needed. Because a number of cheaper, off-the-shelf products are now available to treat neuropathic wounds, custom ankle-foot orthoses are used less often.

Removable Cast Walkers

The effectiveness of removable cast walkers (**Fig. 4**) to reduce pressure at ulcer sites has been shown in several studies to be comparable to that of TCCs.[9,10] Many practitioners consider removable cast walkers to be their preferred offloading device because they are less time-consuming and easier to apply than TCCs, and patients

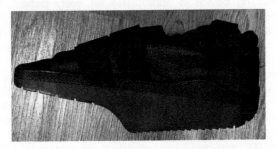

Fig. 2. Wedge shoe.

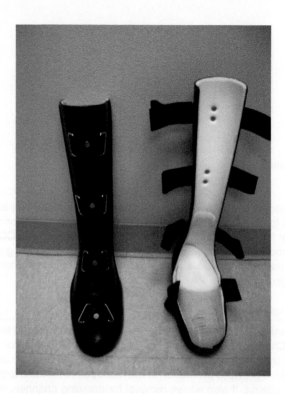

Fig. 3. CROW.

more readily accept them. Wounds can be inspected regularly and treated with advanced wound care products, such as growth factors, electrical stimulation, and other biologically active dressings. Also, the wound and limb can be inspected frequently.

There are additional advantages to using a removable cast walker compared with the TCC. Removable cast walkers are relatively inexpensive and the protective insole can be easily replaced if it shows signs of wear. No special training is required for correct and safe application and they can be easily removed for wound assessment and treatment.[11] It is also possible to modify removable walkers into nonremovable devices by securing the walker with cast material or a nonremovable cable tie; this is known as an instant TCC. If patients cannot remove the walker, the element of forced compliance that makes the TCC attractive is maintained and the outcomes for healing improve to the levels seen with the TCC.[12,13]

No single offloading device is appropriate for every patient. McGuire[14] has suggested a transitional approach to healing and maturing the diabetic foot ulcer that uses the instant TCC for initial pressure management and transitioning to removable devices and shoe-based platforms before the patient is ready for definitive footwear.

In a randomized controlled trial, Armstrong and colleagues[11] compared the effectiveness of TCCs, removable cast walkers, and half-shoes in healing neuropathic foot ulcerations in individuals with diabetes. The percentage of healing at 12 weeks was 89.5% for the TCC, 65.0% for the cast walker, and 58.3% for the half-shoe. When the cast walker is made nonremovable ("instant" total contact cast), the difference between the TCC and cast walker effectively disappears.[15]

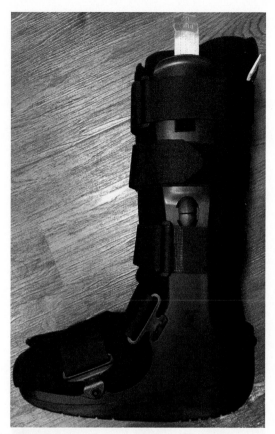

Fig. 4. Removable cast walker.

Total Contact Cast

Use of a TCC (**Figs. 5** and **6**) is considered the gold standard for offloading the foot. TCCs reduce pressure at the ulcer site while still allowing the patient to be ambulatory.[9] Although it is a useful tool, a skilled clinician or technician is required to apply the cast to ensure a proper fit. A poorly fitting cast can cause iatrogenic wounds. A TCC is a modified traditional cast that uses minimal cast padding. This minimal padding is what allows the cast to totally contact the limb, thus limiting potential motion and allowing for equal weight distribution. The cast is molded to the shape and contour of the limb so movement is not possible within the cast. TCCs are generally changed every week to 2 weeks but may need to be replaced more frequently in patients with other comorbidities.

A TCC is one of the most effective ways of treating plantar neuropathic foot ulcers. Numerous studies[10,16–18] have shown that TCCs can heal ulcers in 6 to 8 weeks. The TCC has been shown to decrease pressure to the toes, forefoot, and heel when properly applied.[19] Multiple studies have shown that a TCC heals a higher portion of wounds than topical growth factors, bioengineered tissue, or other alternative methods.[20,21]

Patients who use a TCC are controlled for compliance of use. Although they have the cast applied, the ulceration is protected and the pressure distributed away from

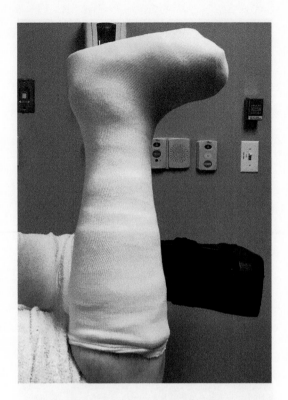

Fig. 5. TCC.

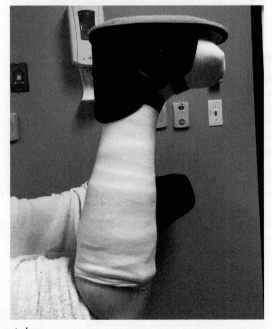

Fig. 6. TCC with cast shoe.

the ulceration and more toward otherwise non–weight-bearing areas, such as the mid-foot.[19] The ulcer is protected with every step the patient takes and compliance is improved, as it is a nonremovable method of offloading. The TCC also reduces the patient's activity level given its weight and size. This in turn decreases stride length, cadence, and pressure at the ulcer site.[9,10] The main disadvantages for patients are from a comfort standpoint; TCCs are heavy, hot, and itchy, and it is not removable, which makes some patients feel trapped.

Recent evidence

A meta-analysis by Elraiyah and colleagues[22] investigated the best available evidence in offloading methods for the diabetic foot ulcer. They identified 19 interventional studies, of which 13 were randomized controlled trials, including data from 1605 patients with diabetic foot ulcers using an offloading method. Their group still demonstrated that TCCs present better evidence to support superior offloading for foot ulcers when compared with a removable cast walker, and other offloading devices. Also, the study by Bus and colleagues[23] demonstrated that removable devices are not as effective as nonremovable devices, but they could be considered for those who cannot tolerate a nonremovable device. In this single-blinded multi-center study, their results show anywhere between 58% and 70% healing of foot ulcers at 12 weeks with 3 different removable offloading devices (bivalved TCC, custom-made ankle high cast shoe, and a prefabricated ankle high forefoot offloading shoe) in their intention-to-treat analysis. Significance was not noted among the 3 devices evaluated.

SUMMARY

Offloading and local wound care continue to be the most essential part of foot ulcer healing. Several methods are available to protect the foot from abnormal pressures. The evidence supports that irremovable devices have a slight edge over removable devices likely due to forced compliance. In general, more restrictive offloading approaches will result in less activity and better wound healing. Offloading needs to be individualized. For many patients, a TCC is not a reasonable option, as their overall health status or personal reasons do not allow for safe or effective use. Therefore, optimizing individual offloading options for each patient is essential.

Reduction of pressure and shear forces on the foot is the single most important, yet most often neglected, aspect of neuropathic ulcer treatment. Offloading therapy is a key part of the treatment plan for diabetic foot ulcers. The goal is to reduce the pressure at the ulcer site while still allowing the patient to remain ambulatory for daily and necessary activities.[6,7] The patient must also be educated that the wound is a result of repetitive pressure and that every step is causing further damage and worsening of the wound. With proper offloading, this damage can be mitigated. Therefore, education is critical to improve compliance with offloading.

REFERENCES

1. Brand P. The diabetic foot. In: Ellenberg M, editor. Diabetes mellitus, theory and practice. Medical Examination; 1983. p. 803–28.
2. Catanzariti AR, Haverstock BD, Grossman JP, et al. Off-loading techniques in the treatment of diabetic plantar neuropathic foot ulceration. Adv Wound Care 1999; 12(9):452–8.
3. Lavery L, Gazewood JD. Assessing the feet of patients with diabetes. J Fam Pract 2000;49(11 Suppl):S9–16.

4. Lavery LA, Armstrong DG, Boulton AJ, et al. Ankle equinus deformity and its relationship to high plantar pressure in a large population with diabetes mellitus. J Am Podiatr Med Assoc 2002;92(9):479–82.

5. Grant WP, Sullivan R, Sonenshine DE, et al. Electron microscopic investigation of the effects of diabetes mellitus on the Achilles tendon. J Foot Ankle Surg 1997; 36(4):272–8 [discussion: 330].

6. Frykberg RG. A summary of guidelines for managing the diabetic foot. Adv Skin Wound Care 2005;18(4):209–14.

7. Lavery LA, Vela SA, Lavery DC, et al. Total contact casts: pressure reduction at ulcer sites and the effect on the contralateral foot. Arch Phys Med Rehabil 1997;78(11):1268–71.

8. Myerson M, Papa J, Eaton K, et al. The total-contact cast for management of neuropathic plantar ulceration of the foot. J Bone Joint Surg Am 1992;74(2): 261–9.

9. Lavery LA, Vela SA, Lavery DC, et al. Reducing dynamic foot pressures in high-risk diabetic subjects with foot ulcerations. A comparison of treatments. Diabetes Care 1996;19(8):818–21.

10. Armstrong DG, Nguyen HC, Lavery LA, et al. Off-loading the diabetic foot wound: a randomized clinical trial. Diabetes Care 2001;24(6):1019–22.

11. Armstrong DG, Lavery LA, Wu S, et al. Evaluation of removable and irremovable cast walkers in the healing of diabetic foot wounds: a randomized controlled trial. Diabetes Care 2005;28(3):551–4.

12. McGuire JB. Pressure redistribution strategies for the diabetic or at-risk foot: part II. Adv Skin Wound Care 2006;19(5):270–7 [quiz: 7–9].

13. Sibbald RG, Woo K, Ayello EA. Increased bacterial burden and infection: the story of NERDS and STONES. Adv Skin Wound Care 2006;19(8):447–61 [quiz: 61–3].

14. McGuire J. Transitional off-loading: an evidence-based approach to pressure redistribution in the diabetic foot. Adv Skin Wound Care 2010;23(4):175–88 [quiz 89–90].

15. Katz IA, Harlan A, Miranda-Palma B, et al. A randomized trial of two irremovable off-loading devices in the management of plantar neuropathic diabetic foot ulcers. Diabetes Care 2005;28(3):555–9.

16. Lavery LA, Armstrong DG, Walker SC. Healing rates of diabetic foot ulcers associated with midfoot fracture due to Charcot's arthropathy. Diabet Med 1997;14(1): 46–9.

17. Sinacore DR. Total contact casting for diabetic neuropathic ulcers. Phys Ther 1996;76(3):296–301.

18. Caputo GM, Ulbrecht JS, Cavanagh PR. The total contact cast: a method for treating neuropathic diabetic ulcers. Am Fam Physician 1997;55(2):605–11, 615-6.

19. Nouman M, Leelasamran W, Chatpun S. Effectiveness of total contact orthosis for plantar pressure redistribution in neuropathic diabetic patients during different walking activities. Foot Ankle Int 2017;38(8):901–8.

20. Veves A, Falanga V, Armstrong DG, et al, Apligraf Diabetic Foot Ulcer Study. Graftskin, a human skin equivalent, is effective in the management of noninfected neuropathic diabetic foot ulcers: a prospective randomized multicenter clinical trial. Diabetes Care 2001;24(2):290–5.

21. Veves A, Sheehan P, Pham HT. A randomized, controlled trial of Promogran (a collagen/oxidized regenerated cellulose dressing) vs standard treatment in the management of diabetic foot ulcers. Arch Surg 2002;137(7):822–7.

22. Elraiyah T, Prutsky G, Domecq JP, et al. A systematic review and meta-analysis of off-loading methods for diabetic foot ulcers. J Vasc Surg 2016;63(2 Suppl): 59S–68S.e1-2.
23. Bus SA, van Netten JJ, Kottink AI, et al. The efficacy of removable devices to off-load and heal neuropathic plantar forefoot ulcers in people with diabetes: a single-blinded multicentre randomised controlled trial. Int Wound J 2018;15(1): 65–74.

A Clinical Review of Diabetic Foot Infections

Cody A. Chastain, MD[a], Nathan Klopfenstein, BSc[a,b], Carlos H. Serezani, PhD[a,b], David M. Aronoff, MD[a,b],*

KEYWORDS

• Diabetic foot infection • Diabetic foot ulcer • Diagnosis • Assessment • Treatment

KEY POINTS

• Diabetic foot infections are common and are usually a consequence of neuropathic ulceration.
• Osteomyelitis is a complication of diabetic foot infections, particularly those associated with longstanding and large foot ulcers.
• Clinical assessment of diabetic foot infections should include the wound, the foot, and the patient as a whole.
• Antimicrobial therapy for diabetic foot infections should be tailored to disease severity, microbial pathogen, and host factors.

INTRODUCTION

Foot infections in persons with diabetes are an important threat to life and limb. This threat is growing, as the number of persons with diabetes has nearly quadrupled in the past 4 decades.[1] It is estimated that diabetic foot infections (DFIs) increase the risk of hospitalization more than 50 times compared with persons without diabetes.[2] DFIs are among the most common diabetes-related cause of hospitalization in the United States, accounting for perhaps 1 in 5 of such hospital admissions.[3] Furthermore, DFIs dramatically increase the likelihood of amputation, to nearly 155 times higher than that for patients without diabetes.[2] Patient anxiety about amputation is extremely high. A recent study found that persons with diabetes and foot disease

Disclosure Statement: The authors have nothing to disclose.
[a] Division of Infectious Diseases, Department of Medicine, Vanderbilt University Medical Center, 1161 21st Avenue South, A-2200 Medical Center North, Nashville, TN 37232-2582, USA;
[b] Department of Pathology, Microbiology and Immunology, Vanderbilt University Medical Center, 1161 21st Avenue South, A-2200 Medical Center North, Nashville, TN 37232-2582, USA
* Corresponding author. Division of Infectious Diseases, Department of Medicine, Vanderbilt University Medical Center, 1161 21st Avenue South, A-2200 Medical Center North, Nashville, TN 37232-2582.
E-mail address: d.aronoff@vumc.org
; @HSerezani (C.H.S.); ; @DMAronoff (D.M.A.)

feared amputation more than death, when compared with persons with diabetes but without foot disease.[4]

The risk of death is significant once infection sets in.[5] Depending on the type of pedal infection, it is estimated that between 1 in 4 to 1 in 8 hospitalized patients will be dead at 1 year.[5] The estimated 5-year mortality of patients with diabetic foot disease (such as ulcers and infections) approaches 50%, a mortality rate that is higher than that for prostate cancer, breast cancer, and Hodgkin lymphoma.[6,7]

Compounding the problem of the rising incidence of DFIs is the increase in antimicrobial resistance (AMR) among common bacterial pathogens found in infected feet.[8] New molecular techniques for the identification of uncultivatable microbes are also broadening our understanding of DFI,[9] while challenging clinicians to think anew about which microbes need to be targeted and which can be ignored.

The purpose of this review was to provide a fresh introduction to the epidemiology of DFIs, summarize key points in their pathogenesis, describe challenges with antimicrobial resistance, review common practices for the diagnosis and management of DFIs (including involvement of bone) and identify important complications of therapy relevant to clinicians.

EPIDEMIOLOGY AND PATHOGENESIS OF DIABETIC FOOT INFECTIONS

Nearly 435 million people are living with diabetes worldwide,[10] and it is estimated that as many as 148 million of those people will a develop foot ulcer (DFU) in their lifetime.[11,12] Because more than 50% of DFUs become infected,[11,13] this translates into nearly 75 million people currently living with diabetes who are likely to develop a foot infection in their lifetime. Broadly defined, DFIs are "any infra-malleolar infection in a person with diabetes mellitus."[14] Common types of DFI are listed in **Table 1**.

There are a number of well-characterized risk factors for foot infection in persons living with diabetes. The primary risk factor for pedal infection in people living with diabetes is an open wound,[2] which is generally a neuropathic DFU.[15,16] Ulcerations precede most foot infections in persons with diabetes[2] and significantly increase the risk of death in this population.[17] In fact, it has been estimated by a prospective study that the risk of developing an infection is >2000 times greater in persons with a foot wound compared with those with intact skin.[2] Apart from a wound itself, other significant risk factors for infection include chronic ulceration (duration more than 30 days), prior lower extremity amputation, the presence of peripheral arterial disease, peripheral neuropathy (described later in this article), renal impairment or transplantation, and walking barefoot.[2,18]

Table 1 Types of diabetic foot infections	
Type of Infection	Involved Structure(s) or Tissue Layer(s)
Paronychia	Soft tissue around a toenail
Cellulitis	Dermis and subcutaneous fat
Myositis	Muscle
Abscess	Inflammatory fluid collection
Necrotizing soft tissue infection	Subcutaneous fat, muscle, and/or fascia
Septic arthritis	Joint space
Tendonitis	Tendon
Osteomyelitis	Bone

The pathogenesis of DFIs is complex and multifactorial. The major processes at play that can result in a DFI are summarized in **Fig. 1**.[14,19] Most DFIs develop because of contiguous spread of bacteria (or, less commonly, fungi) breaching normal skin barriers to establish infection. Less commonly, the soft tissues of the lower extremity can be seeded hematogenously. Contrary to popular belief, most DFIs do not begin as a result of a sudden traumatic event, such as cutting one's foot on a sharp object or stubbing a toe on a foreign object, though such events do occur.

Neuropathic DFUs are the root cause of most DFIs. Thus, the earliest steps in the pathogenesis of DFI is commonly the establishment of a DFU. Neuropathy (autonomic, sensory, and/or motor) is the most critical risk factor driving DFU formation, and this results from chronic, poorly controlled hyperglycemia.[20] Diabetic peripheral neuropathy initially presents as a loss of protective sensation (commonly abbreviated as LOPS), which may not be consciously recognized by the patient. Sensory neuropathy and LOPS allows for improper biomechanics of ambulation (and abnormal load-bearing),[21] which begets osteoarticular damage and deformity (osteoarthropathy), the establishment of callous, and soft tissue necrosis and ulceration.[14,21] Autonomic diabetic neuropathy contributes to skin dryness, increasing the risk for a small crack or wound to occur.[14,21] Peripheral edema of any cause and tinea pedis can also exacerbate skin breakdown and foster cellulitis.

Peripheral vascular disease is a compounding problem in disease pathogenesis. Arterial vascular occlusive disease deprives tissue of needed oxygen, rendering it vulnerable to injury and less capable of healing wounds. It also restricts the arrival of circulating leukocytes to the site of infection.[11] As discussed later in this article, assessing vascular flow, and correcting deficient flow when possible, are important aspects of DFI management and prevention.

Once a wound occurs in a patient with neuropathy, it can become contaminated and colonized with microbes, setting the stage for infection. The risk of skin infection is heightened in persons with diabetes.[22] Although well documented, the cause of this increased susceptibility to infection in the setting of diabetes is not fully understood. Diabetes has been associated with multiple defects in immune defenses.[23]

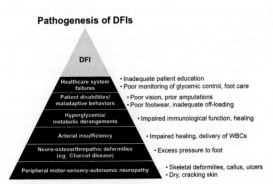

Fig. 1. The pathogenesis of diabetic foot infection (DFI). In this model, DFIs are the result of complex interactions among many preventable factors, including neuropathy, osteoarthropathic bone changes, arterial disease, dysglycemia, maladaptive behaviors, and health care system deficiencies. The primary drivers are noted within the pyramid, whereas pathogenetic features associated with each driver are listed to the side. (*Data from* Lipsky BA, Berendt AR, Deery HG, et al. Diagnosis and treatment of diabetic foot infections. Clin Infect Dis 2004;39(7):885–910; and Lipsky BA, Berendt AR, Deery HG, et al. Diagnosis and treatment of diabetic foot infections. Plast Reconstr Surg 2006;117(7 Suppl):212S–38S.)

Hyperglycemia per se has been suggested as a main culprit of this impaired host defense.[24] Certainly, polymorphonuclear leukocytes (neutrophils) from patients with diabetes have been found to exhibit multiple defects,[25] including impaired chemotactic, phagocytic, and microbicidal activities.[26] Monocytes and macrophages isolated from patients with diabetes have also revealed impaired phagocytic capacity and diminished reactive oxygen species release compared with those from control patients in response to bacterial challenge, resulting in decreased microbial killing.[27] In addition, dendritic cells from persons with diabetes exhibited a diminished ability to migrate to regional lymph nodes, demonstrating impairments in host defense in diabetic patients extend to both innate and adaptive immune responses.[28] Although it is known that hyperglycemia as a result of diabetes is strongly correlated with these impaired immune cell phenotypes, the exact mechanisms by which this occurs remain elusive and are an active area of study.[29,30]

THE IMPORTANCE OF ANTIMICROBIAL RESISTANCE

It has now become apparent that all antibiotics are destined to become ineffective over time.

—Benjamin Lipsky.[31]

Patients with diabetes and foot wounds frequently are treated with antimicrobials, fostering the development of AMR. Globally, AMR is a crisis. It is estimated that by 2050 (unless current trends are reversed), infections due to antibiotic-resistant pathogens will kill more than 10 million people per year worldwide, equating to 1 person dying every 3 seconds.[32,33] Recent studies document the rise in multidrug-resistant pathogens associated with DFIs and their potentially dreadful effects on outcome.[8]

The gram-positive bacterium *Staphylococcus aureus* is a major (if not *the* major) causative agent in nearly all clinical phenotypes of DFI, ranging from mild paronychia to chronic bone infection to life-threatening necrotizing soft tissue infection.[8,34] Methicillin-resistant *S aureus* (MRSA) is now a mainstay of skin and soft tissue infections, particularly those in the feet of persons with diabetes. Compared with hospitalized patients without diabetes, MRSA skin and soft tissue infections in patients with diabetes do not appear to respond as well to antibiotic therapy.[35] There is debate regarding consequences that MRSA infection has on other clinical outcomes in DFI. For example, studies conflict on whether MRSA increases predicted mortality, length of hospital stay, duration of antibiotic therapy, risk for recurrence, or clinical resolution of infection.[36]

The growing threat of AMR in gram-negative bacteria now involves nearly all classes of available agents. Resistance to advanced-generation cephalosporins has emerged in the shape of extended-spectrum beta lactamases and AmpC beta lactamases.[37,38] In addition, a loss of susceptibility to carbapenems has been rapid of late, which occurs as a result of many different mechanisms, including carbapenemase expression. Carbapenem-resistant Enterobacteriaceae are a leading threat to human health. "Pan-resistant" gram-negative bacteria, such as particular isolates of *Pseudomonas* and *Acinetobacter*, are particularly troubling and are being reported in DFIs.[39] There are several risk factors that have been identified predicting the presence of antibiotic-resistant microbes in DFIs and are listed in **Box 1**.

An important driver of AMR in the setting of diabetic foot wounds is biofilm formation, which can provide shielding for microbes against antibiotics, contributing greatly to treatment resistance and persistence.[40,41] Surgical debridement of wounds can be an important traditional therapy for removing or disrupting biofilms. Novel approaches

---

Box 1
Common and important risk factors for antimicrobial-resistant pathogens

Risk factor
Previous use of antibiotics in the past 6 months (especially for the same infection/wound)
Frequent contact with the health care system, including hospitalizations and long-term care facilities
Presence of multiple comorbidities
Prolonged foot wound duration (>30 days)
Chronic infection (eg, osteomyelitis)
Known nasal or rectal carriage (MRSA and gram-negative organisms)
Previous infection with an antibiotic-resistant pathogen

Abbreviation: MRSA, methicillin-resistant *S. aureus.*

Data from Refs.[18,37,92]

---

to combatting biofilms in DFI will gain importance, but their development and application extends beyond the scope of this review.

INITIAL APPROACH TO THE PATIENT WITH DIABETIC FOOT INFECTION

A clinically appropriate and consistent approach to possible DFI is to assess the wound, the foot, and then the patient as a whole. This method is consistent with that outlined by the Infectious Diseases Society of America (IDSA) and the International Working Group on the Diabetic Foot (IWGDF).[42,43] Wound assessment should include evaluation for signs and symptoms of active infection, which may include swelling, induration, erythema, pain, warmth, and/or purulent discharge. The absence of these factors should exclude clinical infection, whereas their presence increases the likelihood of active disease. The involved foot should then be assessed for evidence of distal spread of infection beyond 2 cm from a wound, as well as for other causes of foot inflammation (eg, trauma, fracture, thrombosis, or gout). Furthermore, the involved foot should be assessed for biomechanical, vascular, and neurologic abnormalities that may indicate the underlying risk or cause of a diabetic foot ulcer and/or infection (eg, LOPS). Finally, clinicians should evaluate the whole patient for systemic inflammation, and specifically for ≥ 2 systemic inflammatory response syndrome criteria, such as temperature greater than 38°C or less than 36°C; heart rate greater than 90 beats per minute; respiratory rate greater than 20 breaths per minute or $Paco_2$ less than 32 mm Hg; and white blood cell count greater than 12,000 or less than 4000 cells/μL or 10% immature (band) forms. Although the definition of sepsis has evolved since the prior publication of IDSA and IWGDF guidelines, the application of updated sepsis definitions or utilization of the Sequential (Sepsis-Related) Organ Failure Assessment Score may not be consistently used in practice.[44] As such, clinicians should recognize that the historical criteria for "severe" DFIs correlated with a definition of sepsis, which has now been defined as life-threatening organ dysfunction caused by a dysregulated host response to infection.

Prior classifications devised by the IDSA and IWGDF organize DFI assessments in a similar fashion.[42,43] The IDSA Infection Severity classification system and PEDIS Grade, respectively, are both easy to apply clinically and provide consistent definitions for research use. Clinical presentations may be classified as follows: uninfected (PEDIS Grade 1); mild local infection (PEDIS Grade 2); progressive local, deeper, or complicated infections without systemic inflammation (PEDIS Grade 3); or severe infection with evidence of systemic inflammation (PEDIS Grade 4). A consistent approach to DFI assessment may allow clinical programs to engage multidisciplinary and systematic interventions at multiple levels. Other classification systems are available and may assist with other specific institutional needs.[45]

Once the presence, acuity, and severity of a DFI has been established, medical and surgical resources may be appropriately triaged. For patients with acute, mild infection without complication, empiric antibiotic therapy may be prescribed based on likely microbial pathogens without further evaluation or intervention. For patients with subacute, chronic, or more complicated moderate infections, microbial assessment and aggressive wound management before empiric antibiotic therapy may assist in selecting the appropriate antibiotic as well as duration of treatment. For patients with evidence of severe infection, empiric antimicrobial therapy while urgently coordinating diagnostic and surgical evaluation may be the most prudent course, although this may diminish subsequent microbiologic culture yield.[42,43]

DIAGNOSING OSTEOMYELITIS

Diabetic foot osteomyelitis (DFO) is important to diagnose because it impacts treatment and increases the risk for amputation.[46] DFO almost always results from direct, contiguous extension through an overlying infected chronic ulcer. Hematogenous seeding of bone in the foot is much less common. The diagnosis should be suspected when the overlying ulcer is larger than 2 cm^2, the ulcer extends down to bone, and/or the patient has an erythrocyte sedimentation rate greater than 70 mm/h.[37] A high serum C-reactive protein may also be suggestive of DFO (and useful in monitoring the response to therapy).[47,48] The diagnosis of bone infection should be based on clinical signs of infection and supported by a combination of laboratory, microbiological, and radiological evidence.[46]

The ability of a clinician to probe to bone (PTB) through an ulcer with a blunt metal instrument can be helpful in the initial evaluation of DFO, but this is a controversial subject. In the setting of a high clinical suspicion for infection, a positive PTB test is further suggestive of infection, whereas a negative PTB test is not particularly helpful because of a poor negative predictive value.[37,46] On the other hand, in the setting of a low suspicion for contiguous DFO, a positive PTB test should trigger further evaluation (to increase specificity of the diagnosis), whereas a negative PTB test essentially rules out the diagnosis.[37,46]

Radiographic evaluation for DFO continues to evolve, and excellent reviews of this topic are available.[49,50] The standard plain radiograph of the foot is a good first imaging study, which can assess for the presence of radiopaque foreign bodies, soft tissue gas, osteolytic bone changes, and periosteal elevation.[49] However, it can take weeks for such bone changes to occur following the onset of infection, and these studies lack specificity.[49] At present, reflecting its widespread availability and accuracy, MRI remains the primary imaging modality for investigating DFO.[49] In patients with renal insufficiency, it is acceptable to obtain an MRI without gadolinium contrast, because changes consistent with bone infection (edema) can be observed without contrast. Nuclear medicine studies, including radiolabeled white blood cell scintigraphy (either with ^{99m}Tc-hexamethylpropyleneamineoxime or ^{111}In-oxine), and [^{18}F]fluorodeoxyglucose positron emission tomography/computed tomography are emerging as excellent modalities for diagnosing DFO but are not readily available to many clinicians.[50]

Common radiographic modalities struggle to differentiate midfoot Charcot neuro-osteoarthropathic changes from bone infection.[51] DFO should be highly suspected when radiographic evidence of infection is adjacent to a clinically infected ulcer.[51] DFO in the midfoot without contiguous spread from an adjacent wound is uncommon. When Charcot changes are present, the clinician should consider acute fracture as a likely cause of midfoot erythema, edema, pain, and warmth.

Seeking a specific microbial etiology of bone infection can improve treatment outcomes.[52] Culturing bone is important because bone cultures are often discordant with cultures obtained from overlying soft tissue or sinus tracts.[53–55] An important, albeit small, study reported that medical therapy for DFO was significantly more successful when therapy was guided by bone biopsy as opposed to soft tissue swab culture.[52] Bone biopsy is best performed following an antibiotic-free period of at least 2 weeks, provided the infection is not severe and that the patient does not need urgent antibiotic therapy.[53] Results of a larger study comparing bone culture–directed therapy to soft tissue culture–directed therapy, the Concordance in Diabetic Foot Ulcer Infection study, are eagerly awaited.[55]

EMPIRIC AND DIRECTED ANTIBIOTIC TREATMENT FOR DIABETIC FOOT INFECTION

Once a DFI has been clinically assessed, microbial etiologies and antibiotic treatment options may be considered. Microbiologic assessment should be obtained before initiation of empiric antibiotic therapy if the patient is clinically stable and therapy can be deferred safely.[42,43] The need for antibiotic therapy before surgical debridement may vary depending on the acuity of presentation, the impact of preoperative antibiotic therapy on subsequent interventions, as well as the diagnostic and therapeutic goals of surgical intervention.

Despite the prevalence and impact of DFI, there is a lack of data to support specific antimicrobial approaches. This is in part due to the broad definition of DFI, the variation of anatomic and host settings for infection, as well as the wide spectrum of microbes that may cause infection. Clinical trials that have been performed addressing the treatment of DFI have provided a handful of core observations that support general recommendations; however, additional data are necessary to shape future guidance.[56,57]

The ideal route of antibiotic therapy (ie, oral vs intravenous) for DFI remains controversial. Although topical therapy has theoretic advantages, including direct antibiotic delivery while mitigating systemic toxicity, there are few robust clinical data that support the efficacy of topical antimicrobial treatment; further study in this area may reveal a future, consistent role for topical therapy as a preferred or adjunctive treatment option.[58] As such, oral and intravenous formulations remain the most common administration routes. Although most experts recommend intravenous antibiotic therapy at least initially for severe infections, the duration of intravenous therapy required for optimal outcomes remains uncertain.[42,43] Limited but important literature has demonstrated effective oral antibiotic bioavailability as well as outcomes in skin and soft tissue infections, including osteomyelitis. Although critics have suggested that oral therapy has limited empirical support, there is also a paucity of data to suggest that intravenous antibiotics are superior.[59] Emerging data are promising in that at least some cases of bone and joint infection may be treated equally well by either oral or intravenous therapy.[60,61] Other clinical trial data suggest that oral therapy has at least a partial role after initial intravenous therapy.[62] For mild infections, oral therapy is likely sufficient. For moderate infections, oral therapy alone or a short course of intravenous therapy followed by oral therapy may be appropriate. The optimal approach for severe DFI remains uncertain, and definitive future recommendations will require additional clinical data; in the interim, clinical judgment based on individual patient factors will continue to drive clinical decision making.[42,43]

Acute, mild infections are most commonly attributed to gram-positive organisms including *Staphylococcus* and *Streptococcus*. Empiric antibiotic regimens often include cephalexin, amoxicillin-clavulanate, and clindamycin. Expanding antibiotic spectra of activity to include MRSA as well as gram-negative bacteria may be necessary for DFIs that have failed to respond to prior antibiotic regimens. Patients with unique risk factors predisposing to *Pseudomonas aeruginosa* (ie, exposure to water, puncture wounds, warm climate such as in Africa and Asia) may benefit from empiric therapy addressing this pathogen. Infections that are associated with chronic wounds and/or have failed prior antibiotic treatment courses are more likely to be polymicrobial and may warrant appropriately broadened antimicrobial spectra of activity. Wounds that are necrotic or with fetid odor may include anaerobic pathogens; as such, anaerobic antimicrobial coverage should be included when treating these cases. Patients with severe infections with systemic inflammation may benefit from initial treatment with intravenous therapy including broad antimicrobial spectra of activity, such as vancomycin in combination with a beta-lactam and beta-lactamase inhibitor (eg, ampicillin-sulbactam, piperacillin-tazobactam) or a carbapenem (eg, ertapenem, meropenem). Once a specific microbial pathogen(s) has been identified, antimicrobial therapy should be directed toward that pathogen to reduce unnecessarily broad antimicrobial treatment.[42,43]

DFO is usually a polymicrobial process.[46,53,63,64] Staphylococci (such as *S aureus* and coagulase-negative *Staphylococcus*) and streptococci are commonly involved,[55] whereas in warm climates gram-negative bacteria such as *Escherichia coli* and *Pseudomonas* should be considered.[53] Increasingly, studies suggest that anaerobic bacteria are involved.[64] Thus, anaerobic cultures of bone samples should be performed if at all possible. Empiric and directed treatment for DFO may be selected accordingly.

Once the need for therapy is established, a route is selected, and empiric or directed antimicrobials are prescribed, the duration of antibiotic therapy must be determined. The severity of infection as well as the presence of bone or joint infection are the most important factors to guide providers. Based on guideline recommendations, patients with mild soft tissue infection may be treated with 1 to 2 weeks of therapy. Those with moderate soft tissue infection are suggested to receive 1 to 3 weeks of therapy, whereas those with severe soft tissue infections are suggested to receive 2 to 4 weeks of therapy. The recommended duration of antibiotic therapy in the setting of bone or joint infection is highly dependent on the nature of surgical intervention, ranging from as little as 2 to 5 days when no resident infected tissue is presented after surgery to ≥ 3 months for patients with residual dead bone present with or without surgery.[43] Additional data are necessary to amend these expert recommendations. In patients without necrotic bone or other persistent sources of infection, 6 weeks of therapy is likely appropriate for most cases.[65] The duration of therapy may be adjusted based on clinical response to therapy in some cases; in 1 randomized prospective trial, patients without peripheral arterial disease (PAD) who discontinued antibiotic therapy after signs and symptoms of DFI had resolved did equally well as those who continued antibiotics for the full prescribed duration.[66]

MEDICAL, SURGICAL, AND EMERGING MANAGEMENT OF DIABETIC FOOT INFECTION

Although antibiotic therapy is a cornerstone of DFI treatment, other medical treatments are essential for infection cure, wound healing, and overall patient health. Medical treatment of diabetes mellitus should promote optimal blood glucose management as well as reduce microvascular and macrovascular complications; whereas there are few data to support diabetic control as an essential component of DFI management, it is plausible and remains appropriate for general medical care.[67-69] As noted, PAD is a common comorbid condition of patients with diabetes. Medical treatment of this condition as well as revascularization with endovascular or open surgical techniques may be necessary to provide adequate perfusion for antibiotic delivery and wound healing.[70] Wound off-loading, in the form of diabetic insoles, total contact casts, or other mechanical devices, is an important and often underutilized element of ulcer management.[71] Conservative care can be effective in treating DFI; it is important to note that small, randomized, controlled trials have demonstrated similar outcomes between antibiotic-only and conservative surgery groups in select patients.[72]

Direct wound care and associated surgical intervention remain important for many DFI and DFU treatment plans. Debridement is a key intervention for wound care and healing. Although this may be obtained via sharp debridement or other intensive surgical interventions, topical and other wound care therapies may also assist in wound debridement. In addition, innovative wound care strategies including vacuum-assisted wound closure, hyperbaric oxygen therapy, granulocyte colony-stimulating factor, and novel wound dressings may have increasing roles in DFU as well as DFI management as more robust data become available.[73–77] Despite maximal efforts to manage infection, debride wounds, and revascularize limbs, partial limb amputation may be necessary in cases of severe necrosis, gangrene, or resistant infection.[78–80] Further medical optimization postamputation is critical, as prior DFU and DFI are highly associated with recurrent pathology.[81,82]

COMPLICATIONS OF MEDICAL MANAGEMENT OF DIABETIC FOOT INFECTION

Although antibiotic therapy remains a cornerstone of DFI management, adverse effects and unintended consequences do occur. Direct adverse effects of antibiotic therapy may include drug allergy, gastrointestinal side effects, hematologic side effects, and renal and hepatic toxicity.[83,84] Certain medication, including intravenous vancomycin, require appropriate laboratory monitoring for appropriate dosing as well as for end organ dysfunction (ie, acute kidney injury).[85] Unique drug adverse interactions and adverse effects, such as serotonin syndrome with linezolid or rhabdomyolysis with daptomycin, should be considered and monitored by prescribing providers.[86,87] As previously noted, AMR due to antibiotic exposure has and continues to occur.[88] The emergence of multidrug pathogens as a part of the microbial ecosystem for DFI is both a caution to unnecessary antibiotic prescribing but also an invitation to use advanced agents when necessary. In addition to multidrug resistant pathogens, *Clostridium difficile* infection has emerged as a community and hospital complication in part due to antibiotic exposure.[89] In light of these concerns, it is important for providers to differentiate between uninfected and infected wounds and to select appropriate spectrum and duration of treatment to reduce individual patient as well as public health harm.

THE ROLE OF INFECTIOUS DISEASES SPECIALISTS

It should be noted that health care providers (including pharmacists) with expertise in infectious disease medicine can be an important asset to a team-based approach to diagnosis and management of skin and skin structure infections, including DFI and DFO. In fact, multiple studies have shown, particularly for MRSA infections, that infectious diseases consultation is associated with improved clinical and cost outcomes.[90,91] The appropriate use of antimicrobials, referred to as antimicrobial stewardship, is increasingly important in the era of AMR. Both infectious disease physicians and pharmacists can help reduce inappropriate antibiotic use, avoid complications, and improve outcomes for patients with DFI and DFO.

SUMMARY

The aging of the population and the rise in the prevalence of diabetes are factors driving an increase in the global burden of DFIs. The appropriate clinical approach to the patient with a suspected DFI includes assessment of the infected wound, the associated limb, and the patient as a whole. Bone infection is important to consider in select patients because of its impact on therapy and prognosis. The increasing challenge of AMR compels the need for good cultures of infected sites, appropriate selection of empiric and directed antibiotic therapy, use of all appropriate treatment modalities, as well and coordination among multiple disciplines.

REFERENCES

1. Roglic G. WHO Global report on diabetes: a summary. Int J Noncommun Dis 2016;1(1):3.
2. Lavery LA, Armstrong DG, Wunderlich RP, et al. Risk factors for foot infections in individuals with diabetes. Diabetes Care 2006;29(6):1288–93.
3. Hobizal KB, Wukich DK. Diabetic foot infections: current concept review. Diabet Foot Ankle 2012;3:1–8.
4. Wukich DK, Raspovic KM, Suder NC. Patients with diabetic foot disease fear major lower-extremity amputation more than death. Foot Ankle Spec 2018;11(1): 17–21.
5. Fincke BG, Miller DR, Turpin R. A classification of diabetic foot infections using ICD-9-CM codes: application to a large computerized medical database. BMC Health Serv Res 2010;10(1):192.
6. Armstrong DG, Wrobel J, Robbins JM. Guest Editorial: are diabetes-related wounds and amputations worse than cancer? Int Wound J 2007;4(4):286–7.
7. Robbins JM, Strauss G, Aron D, et al. Mortality rates and diabetic foot ulcers: is it time to communicate mortality risk to patients with diabetic foot ulceration? J Am Podiatr Med Assoc 2008;98(6):489–93.
8. Saltoglu N, Ergonul O, Tulek N, et al. Influence of multidrug resistant organisms on the outcome of diabetic foot infection. Int J Infect Dis 2018;70:10–4.
9. Malone M, Johani K, Jensen SO, et al. Next generation DNA sequencing of tissues from infected diabetic foot ulcers. EBioMedicine 2017;21:142–9.
10. GBD 2015 Disease and Injury Incidence and Prevalence Collaborators. Global, regional, and national incidence, prevalence, and years lived with disability for 310 diseases and injuries, 1990-2015: a systematic analysis for the Global Burden of Disease Study 2015. Lancet 2016;388(10053):1545–602.
11. Armstrong DG, Boulton AJ, Bus SA. Diabetic foot ulcers and their recurrence. N Engl J Med 2017;376(24):2367–75.
12. Lazzarini PA, Pacella RE, Armstrong DG, et al. Diabetes-related lower-extremity complications are a leading cause of the global burden of disability. Diabet Med 2018;35(9):1297–9.
13. Prompers L, Huijberts M, Apelqvist J, et al. High prevalence of ischaemia, infection and serious comorbidity in patients with diabetic foot disease in Europe. Baseline results from the Eurodiale study. Diabetologia 2007;50(1):18–25.
14. Lipsky BA, Berendt AR, Deery HG, et al, Infectious Diseases Society of America. Diagnosis and treatment of diabetic foot infections. Clin Infect Dis 2004;885–910.
15. Reiber GE, Vileikyte L, Boyko EJ, et al. Causal pathways for incident lower-extremity ulcers in patients with diabetes from two settings. Diabetes Care 1999;22(1):157–62.

16. Noor S, Khan RU, Ahmad J. Understanding diabetic foot infection and its management. Diabetes Metab Syndr 2017;11(2):149–56.
17. Walsh JW, Hoffstad OJ, Sullivan MO, et al. Association of diabetic foot ulcer and death in a population-based cohort from the United Kingdom. Diabet Med 2016; 33(11):1493–8.
18. Nikoloudi M, Eleftheriadou I, Tentolouris A, et al. Diabetic foot infections: update on management. Curr Infect Dis Rep 2018;20(10):40.
19. Lipsky BA, Berendt AR, Deery HG, et al, Infectious Diseases Society of America. Diagnosis and treatment of diabetic foot infections. Plast Reconstr Surg 2006; 117(7 Suppl):212S–38S.
20. Frykberg RG, Cook JJ, Simonson DC. Epidemiology and health care cost of diabetic foot problems. In: Veves A, Giurini JM, Guzman RJ, editors. The Diabetic Foot. Cham (Switzerland): Humana Press; 2018. p. 3–17.
21. Ulbrecht JS, Cavanagh PR, Caputo GM. Foot problems in diabetes: an overview. Clin Infect Dis 2004;39(Supplement_2):S73–82.
22. Joshi N, Caputo GM, Weitekamp MR, et al. Infections in patients with diabetes mellitus. N Engl J Med 1999;341(25):1906–12.
23. Geerlings SE, Hoepelman AI. Immune dysfunction in patients with diabetes mellitus (DM). FEMS Immunol Med Microbiol 1999;26(3–4):259–65.
24. Jafar N, Edriss H, Nugent K. The effect of short-term hyperglycemia on the innate immune system. Am J Med Sci 2016;351(2):201–11.
25. Delamaire M, Maugendre D, Moreno M, et al. Impaired leucocyte functions in diabetic patients. Diabet Med 1997;14(1):29–34.
26. Alba-Loureiro TC, Munhoz CD, Martins JO, et al. Neutrophil function and metabolism in individuals with diabetes mellitus. Braz J Med Biol Res 2007;40(8): 1037–44.
27. Turina M, Fry DE, Polk HC Jr. Acute hyperglycemia and the innate immune system: clinical, cellular, and molecular aspects. Crit Care Med 2005;33(7):1624–33.
28. Dejani NN, Brandt SL, Piñeros A, et al. Topical prostaglandin E analog restores defective dendritic cell-mediated Th17 host defense against methicillin-resistant Staphylococcus aureus in the skin of diabetic mice. Diabetes 2016; 65(12):3718–29.
29. Domingueti CP, Dusse LM, Carvalho MD, et al. Diabetes mellitus: the linkage between oxidative stress, inflammation, hypercoagulability and vascular complications. J Diabetes Complications 2016;30(4):738–45.
30. Wada J, Makino H. Innate immunity in diabetes and diabetic nephropathy. Nat Rev Nephrol 2016;12(1):13–26.
31. Lipsky BA. Diabetic foot infections: current treatment and delaying the 'post-antibiotic era'. Diabetes Metab Res Rev 2016;32:246–53.
32. Goff DA, Kullar R, Goldstein EJC, et al. A global call from five countries to collaborate in antibiotic stewardship: united we succeed, divided we might fail. Lancet Infect Dis 2017;17(2):e56–63.
33. O'Neill J. Antimicrobial resistance: tackling a crisis for the health and wealth of nations. London (United Kingdom): Review on Antimicrobial Resistance; 2017.
34. U, kay I, Gariani K, Dubois-Ferrière V, et al. Diabetic foot infections: recent literature and cornerstones of management. Curr Opin Infect Dis 2016;29(2):145–52.
35. Lipsky BA, Itani KM, Weigelt JA, et al. The role of diabetes mellitus in the treatment of skin and skin structure infections caused by methicillin-resistant Staphylococcus aureus: results from three randomized controlled trials. Int J Infect Dis 2011;15(2):e140–6.

36. Zenelaj B, Bouvet C, Lipsky BA, et al. Do diabetic foot infections with methicillin-resistant *Staphylococcus aureus* differ from those with other pathogens? Int J Low Extrem Wounds 2014;13(4):263–72.

37. LaSalvia MT, Karchmer AW. Microbiology and treatment of diabetic foot infection. In: Veves A, Giurini JM, Guzman RJ, editors. The Diabetic Foot. Cham (Switzerland): Humana Press; 2018. p. 267–79.

38. Xie X, Bao Y, Ni L, et al. Bacterial profile and antibiotic resistance in patients with diabetic foot ulcer in Guangzhou, Southern China: focus on the differences among different Wagner's Grades, IDSA/IWGDF Grades, and ulcer types. Int J Endocrinol 2017;2017:8694903.

39. Sekhar SM, Vyas N, Unnikrishnan M, et al. Antimicrobial susceptibility pattern in diabetic foot ulcer: a pilot study. Ann Med Health Sci Res 2014;4(5):742–5.

40. Vatan A, Saltoglu N, Yemisen M, et al. Association between biofilm and multi/extensive drug resistance in diabetic foot infection. Int J Clin Pract 2018;72(3):e13060.

41. Mottola C, Matias CS, Mendes JJ, et al. Susceptibility patterns of *Staphylococcus aureus* biofilms in diabetic foot infections. BMC Microbiol 2016;16(1):119.

42. Lipsky BA, Aragón-Sánchez J, Diggle M, et al. IWGDF guidance on the diagnosis and management of foot infections in persons with diabetes. Diabetes Metab Res Rev 2016;32(Suppl 1):45–74.

43. Lipsky BA, Berendt AR, Cornia PB, et al. 2012 Infectious Diseases Society of America clinical practice guideline for the diagnosis and treatment of diabetic foot infections. Clin Infect Dis 2012;54(12):e132–73.

44. Singer M, Deutschman CS, Seymour CW, et al. The third international consensus definitions for sepsis and septic shock (Sepsis-3). JAMA 2016;315(8):801–10.

45. Game F. Classification of diabetic foot ulcers. Diabetes Metab Res Rev 2016;32(Suppl 1):186–94.

46. Giurato L, Meloni M, Izzo V, et al. Osteomyelitis in diabetic foot: a comprehensive overview. World J Diabetes 2017;8(4):135–42.

47. van Asten SA, Jupiter DC, Mithani M, et al. Erythrocyte sedimentation rate and C-reactive protein to monitor treatment outcomes in diabetic foot osteomyelitis. Int Wound J 2017;14(1):142–8.

48. Victoria van Asten SA, Geradus Peters EJ, Xi Y, et al. The role of biomarkers to diagnose diabetic foot osteomyelitis. A meta-analysis. Curr Diabetes Rev 2016;12(4):396–402.

49. Peterson N, Widnall J, Evans P, et al. Diagnostic imaging of diabetic foot disorders. Foot Ankle Int 2017;38(1):86–95.

50. Lauri C, Tamminga M, Glaudemans AWJM, et al. Detection of osteomyelitis in the diabetic foot by imaging techniques: a systematic review and meta-analysis comparing MRI, white blood cell scintigraphy, and FDG-PET. Diabetes Care 2017;40(8):1111–20.

51. Rogers LC, Frykberg RG. The diabetic charcot foot. In: Veves A, Giurini JM, Guzman RJ, editors. The Diabetic Foot. Cham (Switzerland): Humana Press; 2018. p. 391–413.

52. Senneville E, Lombart A, Beltrand E, et al. Outcome of diabetic foot osteomyelitis treated nonsurgically: a retrospective cohort study. Diabetes Care 2008;31(4):637–42.

53. Senneville E, Robineau O. Treatment options for diabetic foot osteomyelitis. Expert Opin Pharmacother 2017;18(8):759–65.

54. Vris A, Massa E, Ahluwalia R, et al. Primary results of bone biopsies in outpatients with neuropathic ulcers: comparison with wound swabs and superficial tissue samples. Foot & Ankle Orthopaedics 2017;2(3). 2473011417S000078.

55. Nelson A, Wright-Hughes A, Backhouse MR, et al. CODIFI (Concordance in Diabetic Foot Ulcer Infection): a cross-sectional study of wound swab versus tissue sampling in infected diabetic foot ulcers in England. BMJ Open 2018;8(1): e019437.

56. Selva Olid A, Solà I, Barajas-Nava LA, et al. Systemic antibiotics for treating diabetic foot infections. Cochrane Database Syst Rev 2015;(9):CD009061.

57. Tchero H, Kangambega P, Noubou L, et al. Antibiotic therapy of diabetic foot infections: a systematic review of randomized controlled trials. Wound Repair Regen 2018;26(5):381–91.

58. Dumville JC, Lipsky BA, Hoey C, et al. Topical antimicrobial agents for treating foot ulcers in people with diabetes. Cochrane Database Syst Rev 2017;6: CD011038.

59. Spellberg B, Lipsky BA. Systemic antibiotic therapy for chronic osteomyelitis in adults. Clin Infect Dis 2012;54(3):393–407.

60. Li HK, Scarborough M, Zambellas R, et al. Oral versus intravenous antibiotic treatment for bone and joint infections (OVIVA): study protocol for a randomised controlled trial. Trials 2015;16:583.

61. Scarborough M, Li HK, Rombach I, et al. Oral versus intravenous antibiotics for the treatment of bone and joint infection (OVIVA): a multicentre randomized controlled trial in Orthopaedic Proceedings. 2017: The British Editorial Society of Bone & Joint Surgery.

62. Schaper NC, Dryden M, Kujath P, et al. Efficacy and safety of IV/PO moxifloxacin and IV piperacillin/tazobactam followed by PO amoxicillin/clavulanic acid in the treatment of diabetic foot infections: results of the RELIEF study. Infection 2013;41(1):175–86.

63. Johani K, Fritz BG, Bjarnsholt T, et al. Understanding the microbiome of diabetic foot osteomyelitis: insights from molecular and microscopic approaches. Clin Microbiol Infect 2019;25(3):332–9.

64. van Asten SA, La Fontaine J, Peters EJ, et al. The microbiome of diabetic foot osteomyelitis. Eur J Clin Microbiol Infect Dis 2016;35(2):293–8.

65. Tone A, Nguyen S, Devemy F, et al. Six-week versus twelve-week antibiotic therapy for nonsurgically treated diabetic foot osteomyelitis: a multicenter open-label controlled randomized study. Diabetes Care 2015;38(2):302–7.

66. Chu Y, Wang C, Zhang J, et al. Can we stop antibiotic therapy when signs and symptoms have resolved in diabetic foot infection patients? Int J Low Extrem Wounds 2015;14(3):277–83.

67. Fullerton B, Jeitler K, Seitz M, et al. Intensive glucose control versus conventional glucose control for type 1 diabetes mellitus. Cochrane Database Syst Rev 2014;(2):CD009122.

68. Paneni F, Luscher TF. Cardiovascular protection in the treatment of type 2 diabetes: a review of clinical trial results across drug classes. Am J Med 2017; 130(6S):S18–29.

69. Ueki K, Sasako T, Okazaki Y, et al. Effect of an intensified multifactorial intervention on cardiovascular outcomes and mortality in type 2 diabetes (J-DOIT3): an open-label, randomised controlled trial. Lancet Diabetes Endocrinol 2017;5(12): 951–64.

70. Hinchliffe RJ, Brownrigg JR, Andros G, et al. Effectiveness of revascularization of the ulcerated foot in patients with diabetes and peripheral artery disease: a systematic review. Diabetes Metab Res Rev 2016;32(Suppl 1):136–44.

71. Fife CE, Carter MJ, Walker D, et al. Diabetic foot ulcer off-loading: the gap between evidence and practice. Data from the US Wound Registry. Adv Skin Wound Care 2014;27(7):310–6.

72. Lazaro-Martinez JL, Aragon-Sanchez J, Garcia-Morales E. Antibiotics versus conservative surgery for treating diabetic foot osteomyelitis: a randomized comparative trial. Diabetes Care 2014;37(3):789–95.

73. Fedorko L, Bowen JM, Jones W, et al. Hyperbaric oxygen therapy does not reduce indications for amputation in patients with diabetes with nonhealing ulcers of the lower limb: a prospective, double-blind, randomized controlled clinical trial. Diabetes Care 2016;39(3):392–9.

74. Huang ET, Mansouri J, Murad MH, et al. A clinical practice guideline for the use of hyperbaric oxygen therapy in the treatment of diabetic foot ulcers. Undersea Hyperb Med 2015;42(3):205–47.

75. Liu Z, Dumville JC, Hinchliffe RJ, et al. Negative pressure wound therapy for treating foot wounds in people with diabetes mellitus. Cochrane Database Syst Rev 2018;(10):CD010318.

76. Cruciani M, Lipsky BA, Mengoli C, et al. Granulocyte-colony stimulating factors as adjunctive therapy for diabetic foot infections. Cochrane Database Syst Rev 2013;(8):CD006810.

77. Edmonds M, Lázaro-Martínez JL, Alfayate-García JM, et al. Sucrose octasulfate dressing versus control dressing in patients with neuroischaemic diabetic foot ulcers (Explorer): an international, multicentre, double-blind, randomised, controlled trial. Lancet Diabetes Endocrinol 2018;6(3):186–96.

78. Callahan D, Keeley J, Alipour H, et al. Predictors of severity in diabetic foot infections. Ann Vasc Surg 2016;33:103–8.

79. Uysal S, Arda B, Taşbakan MI, et al. Risk factors for amputation in patients with diabetic foot infection: a prospective study. Int Wound J 2017;14(6):1219–24.

80. Zhan LX, Branco BC, Armstrong DG, et al. The Society for Vascular Surgery lower extremity threatened limb classification system based on Wound, Ischemia, and foot Infection (WIfI) correlates with risk of major amputation and time to wound healing. J Vasc Surg 2015;61(4):939–44.

81. Dubský M, Jirkovská A, Bem R, et al. Risk factors for recurrence of diabetic foot ulcers: prospective follow-up analysis in the Eurodiale subgroup. Int Wound J 2013;10(5):555–61.

82. Örneholm H, Apelqvist J, Larsson J, et al. Recurrent and other new foot ulcers after healed plantar forefoot diabetic ulcer. Wound Repair Regen 2017;25(2):309–15.

83. Keller SC, Dzintars K, Gorski LA, et al. Antimicrobial agents and catheter complications in outpatient parenteral antimicrobial therapy. Pharmacotherapy 2018;38(4):476–81.

84. Keller SC, Williams D, Gavgani M, et al. Rates of and risk factors for adverse drug events in outpatient parenteral antimicrobial therapy. Clin Infect Dis 2018;66(1):11–9.

85. Schrank GM, Wright SB, Branch-Elliman W, et al. A retrospective analysis of adverse events among patients receiving daptomycin versus vancomycin during outpatient parenteral antimicrobial therapy. Infect Control Hosp Epidemiol 2018;39(8):947–54.

86. Papadopoulos S, Ball AM, Liewer SE, et al. Rhabdomyolysis during therapy with daptomycin. Clin Infect Dis 2006;42(12):e108–10.
87. Wigen CL, Goetz MB. Serotonin syndrome and linezolid. Clin Infect Dis 2002; 34(12):1651–2.
88. Chatterjee A, Modarai M, Naylor NR, et al. Quantifying drivers of antibiotic resistance in humans: a systematic review. Lancet Infect Dis 2018;18(12):e368–78.
89. McDonald LC, Gerding DN, Johnson S, et al. Clinical practice guidelines for *Clostridium difficile* infection in adults and children: 2017 update by the infectious diseases Society of America (IDSA) and Society for health care epidemiology of America (SHEA). Clin Infect Dis 2018;66(7):e1–48.
90. Schmitt S, McQuillen DP, Nahass R, et al. Infectious diseases specialty intervention is associated with decreased mortality and lower healthcare costs. Clin Infect Dis 2013;58(1):22–8.
91. Vogel M, Schmitz RP, Hagel S, et al. Infectious disease consultation for Staphylococcus aureus bacteremia–a systematic review and meta-analysis. J Infect 2016;72(1):19–28.
92. Kwon KT, Armstrong DG. Microbiology and antimicrobial therapy for diabetic foot infections. Infect Chemother 2018;50(1):11–20.

Dressings, Topical Therapy, and Negative Pressure Wound Therapy

Leland Jaffe, DPM, CWSP[a],*, Stephanie C. Wu, DPM, MSc[b]

KEYWORDS

• Wounds • Dressings • Topical therapy • Negative pressure wound therapy

KEY POINTS

• Proper assessment and management of the wound-bed environment through the use of appropriate dressings can facilitate wound healing.
• The use of negative pressure wound therapy (NPWT) can accelerate wound healing through the use of subatmospheric pressure. Multiple product designs exist to allow for application of NPWT in various clinical scenarios.
• Failure of the wound to progress through the stages of wound healing should prompt the clinician to consider an alternative treatment plan including the use of advanced topical wound therapies.

INTRODUCTION

Wound management has become a significant medical necessity within the health care system because of the epidemic of chronic diseases. Chronic wounds present a significant psychological, physical, and financial burden for patients. Chronic wounds are defined as those that do not progress through the stages of healing in an organized fashion to create structural integrity of the skin.[1] It has been estimated that about 1% to 2% of the general population will develop a chronic wound during their lifetime,[2] including 6.5 million patients in the United States.[3] The economic implications of this epidemic are also growing rapidly because of the aging population as well as the increased prevalence of chronic diseases such as diabetes mellitus, heart

Disclosure Statement: No financial disclosures or conflicts of interest to report.
[a] Department of Medicine and Radiology, Dr William M. Scholl College of Podiatric Medicine at Rosalind Franklin University, 3333 Green Bay Road, North Chicago, IL 60064, USA;
[b] Department of Podiatric Surgery and Applied Biomechanics, Center for Stem Cell and Regenerative Medicine, Center for Lower Extremity Ambulatory Research (CLEAR), Dr William M. Scholl College of Podiatric Medicine at Rosalind Franklin University of Medicine and Science, 3333 Green Bay Road, North Chicago, IL 60064, USA
* Corresponding author.
E-mail address: leland.jaffe@rosalindfranklin.edu

disease, and obesity. In addition it is estimated that in excess of 25 billion dollars are spent annually in the United States for the treatment of chronic wounds,[4] and this number is expected to continue to increase.

Proper dressing selection for a wound focuses on maintaining adequate moisture level, minimizing bacterial bioburden, controlling exudate, and temperature regulation. Observance to these fundamental principles assists with the progression toward granulation tissue formation and eventual epithelialization and closure of the wound (**Box 1**).

An intact epithelium is our body's greatest barrier to the loss of fluids. The wound-bed tissue is at significant risk of desiccation following loss of the stratum corneum, placing the wound at risk of delayed progression through the stages of healing.[5] A moist wound environment has been demonstrated to improve wound healing by assisting with cellular migration and granulation tissue formation, and reducing infection rates.[6] The wound bed can range from accumulating desiccated nonviable tissue to excessive moisture buildup and periwound maceration, both of which will compromise the formation of healthy granular tissue and eventual skin epithelialization. Chronic wound fluid is noted to have abundant matrix metalloproteinases (MMPs) and other proinflammatory cytokines,[7,8] prolonging the inflammatory stage of wound healing. By contrast, too little moisture can prevent cellular activity and keratinocyte migration across the wound surface.[5] Adequate moisture balance is essential to facilitate the normal cellular activity leading to wound closure. The type and quantity of the wound exudate will determine the specific needs of the wounds. Wounds that are dry require a hydrating dressing such as a hydrogel, Manuka honey, or a hydrocolloid dressing. In recent studies comparing the efficacy of several dressings in the healing of diabetic foot ulcers (DFUs), hydrogel dressings along with amniotic membranes were noted as the preferred solutions for healing DFUs.[9,10] Meta-analyses have confirmed that the use of hydrocolloids in comparison with standard gauze dressing results in accelerated wound healing.[11,12] Excessive moisture, by contrast, will require an absorptive dressing including an alginate, hydrofiber, or foam.[13]

The TIME (Tissue, Infection/Inflammation, Moisture, Edge of wound) principle was introduced to wound-care clinicians in 2003 as a tool to assess for proper wound-healing progression. This form of wound assessment allows the clinician to objectively and systematically evaluate the environment of the wound bed. Adherence to the

---

Box 1
Features of an ideal wound dressing

- Facilitate a moist environment
- Absorb excess exudate
- Prevent desiccation of the wound (donates moistures in dry wounds)
- Protect the periwound tissue
- Maintain a warm environment
- Minimize bacterial bioburden (resistant to microorganisms)
- Minimize or eliminate pain
- Cost-effective
- Eliminate odor
- Eliminate dead space

TIME principles allows for critical continual evaluation of the physiologic needs of the wound bed through the use of topical dressings. Proper wound management involves optimizing the wound bed to facilitate wound closure, which is accomplished via the use of primary and secondary dressings. The primary dressing is applied directly to the wound surface and the secondary dressing is applied to either bolster the primary dressing or provide a therapeutic function. Dressings are organized categorically based on their therapeutic effect on the wound bed and periwound tissue. As wounds progress through the predictable stages of healing (hemostasis, inflammation, proliferation, remodeling), the physiologic needs of the wound may evolve. Clinicians should continue to evaluate for specific considerations regarding wound assessment including the amount of exudate, the depth, the tissue noted in the base of the wound, and the location of the wound.

An effective topical wound dressing is designed to maintain a healthy, physiologic level of moisture, facilitate autolytic debridement through the activity of endogenous enzymes, improve granular tissue formation, and enhance bacterial bioburden management.[14] Therefore, based on the needs of the wound bed, topical dressings can range from moisture-donating, moisture-absorptive, or moisture-retention materials. A moist wound bed may be maintained with the use of occlusive, semiocclusive, absorptive, or hydrating materials. Clinical indications and instructions for clinical use of various types of wound dressings are discussed in **Table 1**.

Topical Antimicrobial Dressings

Given that 60% to 90% of chronic wounds have biofilm,[32] and a biofilm may be reestablished within 3 days following a wound debridement,[32,33] proper wound-bed management and dressing selection is critical to deterring this biofilm reformation. Dressings impregnated with silver, cadexomer iodine, honey, and polyhexamethylene biguanide (PHMB) have all been advocated for the management of wounds containing biofilm[32] (**Table 2**).

TOPICAL WOUND THERAPIES

Wounds should proceed in an unimpeded fashion through the stages of healing. If wounds fail to progress as expected despite an appreciation and adherence to the fundamental principles of wound healing, more advanced topical therapies may be indicated. A meta-analysis published in *Diabetes Care* demonstrated that 24% of DFUs healed at 12 weeks and 31% healed at 20 weeks' duration.[44] In 2003, Sheehan and colleagues[45] determined that the percent change in wound area of DFU at 4 weeks is a strong predictor of complete healing at 12 weeks. In this study it was determined that if DFU did not reduce by 53% at 4 weeks' duration, the healing rate at 12 weeks was 9%. These studies have since been replicated and reproduced, and demonstrate that a failure to achieve an acceptable initial progression of wound closure should prompt the provider to consider advanced topical wound therapies. Topical wound therapies are available as topical growth factors, placental/umbilical cord tissue allograft, acellular dermal matrices, and cell-based therapies. The clinical indications and instructions for clinical use of these therapies are discussed in **Table 3**.

NEGATIVE PRESSURE WOUND THERAPY

Negative pressure wound therapy (NPWT) is a noninvasive wound-management system that uses controlled, localized, subatmospheric pressure to promote healing in chronic and acute wounds. NPWT has been found to assist with promotion of

Table 1
Wound-care dressings

Description of Product	Indications	Contraindications	Instructions for Clinical Use
Contact layer dressings • Petroleum, silicone, polyethylene, or lipidocolloid based • Nonadherent • Semiocclusive • Porous to facilitate exudate removal • Conforms to the shape of the wound • Prevents desiccation by adding moisture to the wound bed[15]	• Partial or full-thickness wounds • Placement on incisions • Overlying split-thickness skin grafts • Overlying bioengineered alternative tissues (BATs) • Placed on donor sites • Atraumatic, painless removal of dressing	• None	• Apply directly to wound bed • Secondary dressing or topical medication placed on contact layer • Indicated to be changed weekly
Hydrogels • Composed of hydrophilic crosslinked polymers that are 80%–90% water[16] or glycerin based • Nonadherent • Facilitate autolytic debridement • Absorb minute amounts of exudate by swelling • Primarily used to donate moisture to the wound surface	• Partial or full-thickness wounds • Dry wounds with minimal exudate	• Third-degree burns • Wound with moderate to severe exudate	• Apply to wound base and use appropriate secondary dressing • Daily applications • Not to be used as a wound filler

Dressing	Uses	Contraindications	Application
Hydrocolloids • Contain an inner self-adhesive layer and a gel-forming agent such as gelatin or sodium carboxymethylcellulose • Inner layer of the hydrocolloid is laminated on a foam or film, typically composed of polyurethane • Absorb exudate and swell to form a gel on the wound bed • Promote autolytic debridement • Create barrier to protect from pathogens	• Partial or full-thickness wounds • Minimal to moderately exudative wounds • Granular or necrotic wound beds	• Third-degree burns • Infected wounds • Eschar	• Apply directly to wound surface • Hydrocolloid placed 2.5–5 cm onto periwound tissue • Dressing changed every 3–5 d pending amount of exudate
Foam dressings • Absorptive dressing • Open-cell polyurethane material • Hydrophilic properties allow absorption of exudate • Atraumatic/painless during dressing changes	• Partial or full-thickness wounds • Moderate to severely exudative wounds • Granular or nongranular wound beds • Reduces shear in pressure skin injuries[17] • Protect wounds with friable periwound tissue	• Third-degree burns • Ischemic arterial wounds with eschar wound base • Wounds with dry/necrotic wound beds • Tunneling wounds	• Used as a primary or secondary wound dressing • Frequency of dressing change will depend of the quantity of exudate, ranging from daily to once weekly
Alginate dressings • Derived from fibers of brown seaweed • Highly absorbent • Convert to a viscous, hydrophilic gel when calcium and sodium salts within the dressing interact with exudate from the wound, providing a moist wound environment • Nonadherent because of gel-forming nature • Hemostatic properties[19] • Provide autolytic debridement	• Partial to full-thickness wounds • Moderate to heavily exudative wounds • Placed within sinus tracks and tunneling wounds	• Dry wounds with minimal exudate • Third-degree burns • Wounds with necrotic tissue present, as no moisture is donated to the wound surface	• Applied daily to weekly depending on the quantity of exudate • Apply appropriate secondary dressing overlying alginate • May be used as packing into tunneling wounds

(continued on next page)

Table 1
(*continued*)

Description of Product	Indications	Contraindications	Instructions for Clinical Use
Hydrofiber dressings • Derived from carboxymethylcellulose • Absorption of copious exudate • Form hydrophilic gelatinous substances that adapt to the wound contour[20] • Facilitate moist wound-healing environment • Nonadherent • Facilitate autolytic wound debridement, granulation tissue formation, and wound epithelialization[21]	• Partial to full-thickness wounds • Moderate to heavy exudative wounds	• Dry wounds with minimal exudate	• Change dressing every 24–48 h pending amount of exudate • Apply appropriate secondary dressing to secure hydrofiber into place
Collagen dressings • Bovine, porcine, and ovine sources • Available in sheet, gel, or powder forms • Bioabsorbable • Chemoattractant for cells involved in wound healing • Inactivate some MMPs, elastase,[22,23] decreasing the level of inflammatory mediators[24,25] • Scaffold to increase collagen production • Bacteriostatic properties in vitro[26] • Silver-impregnated versions available[27] • Increase rate of epithelialization,[28] and accelerate wound closure in patients with recalcitrant wounds[29–31]	• Full-thickness wounds • Wounds with minimal to moderate exudate • Uninfected wounds	• Sensitivity to the tissue of origin (bovine, porcine, ovine)	• Apply to wound bed and secure with secondary dressing • Frequency of dressing change varies based on product and quantity of exudate

Table 2
Antimicrobial topical wound-care therapies

Description of Product	Indications	Contraindications	Instructions for Clinical Use
0.9% Cadexomer iodine • Contains 0.9% iodine • Functions as an antimicrobial agent through its disruption of the bacterial lipid membrane and inhibition of protein synthesis[37,38] • As exudate is absorbed, iodine is slowly released from the dressing, exerting its antiseptic effect[39] • Nontoxic to fibroblasts	• High capacity for absorbing exudate; each gram absorbs 3 mL of exudate • Partial or full-thickness wounds • Critically colonized to infected wounds • Methicillin-resistant *Staphylococcus aureus* (MRSA)	• Allergy to iodine • Hashimoto thyroiditis • Graves disease	• Frequency of application every 24–72 h • Color change from brown to yellow/gray indicates the need for dressing change
Manuka honey • As honey interacts with wound exudate, hydrogen peroxide is produced, creating a broad-spectrum antimicrobial effect[42] • Also functions by eliminating water from bacterial cells, causing lysis of these cells[43] • Promotes autolytic debridement • Anti-inflammatory	• Diabetic, venous, arterial, and pressure ulcers • First- and second-degree burns • Provides a moist wound-healing environment • Light to moderate exudative wounds	• Bee stings	• Available as a hydrogel, hydrocolloid, or alginate • Dressing change protocol varies based on dressing

(continued on next page)

Table 2
(continued)

Description of Product	Indications	Contraindications	Instructions for Clinical Use
Silver dressings and topicals • Antiseptic, anti-inflammatory, with broad-spectrum antimicrobial activity[34] • Silver cations exert antimicrobial effect by blocking cellular respiration and disturbing bacterial cell membranes • Silver can also denature bacteria DNA and RNA, preventing cell replication[35] • Activity against MRSA and vancomycin-resistant *Enterococcus* (VRE)	• Reduces bacterial bioburden	• Allergy to silver • Use with caution in the management of diabetic wounds, owing to a cytotoxic effect to dermal fibroblasts[36]	• Method of silver ion delivery varies by dressing type • Dressing change protocol varies based on dressing
PHMB Products • PHMB has a positively charged structure that binds to the negative charge of the bacterial cell membrane, disrupting the integrity of the bacteria[40] • Efficacy on both planktonic and sessile (biofilm) bacterial colonies[41] • Antiseptic • Noncytotoxic • Not irritating to viable skin • Activity against MRSA, VRE, fungi	• Reduces bacterial bioburden	• None	• Dressing change protocol varies based on dressing

Table 3
Advanced topical wound-care therapies

Category of Products	Description of Product	Clinical Indications	Instructions for Clinical Use
Topical growth factor therapy	• Platelet-derived growth factor (PDGF) • PDGF recruits and stimulates fibroblast proliferation, promoting granulation tissue formation[46]	• Lower extremity neuropathic diabetic ulcerations • Indicated for wounds that extend to the subcutaneous tissue or deeper • No evidence to support use on joints, tendons, ligaments, or bone	• Applied once daily to wound bed with moistened gauze dressing covering the area • Contraindicated in patients with neoplasm at the side of application • Contraindicated in patients with allergy to parabens
Acellular extracellular matrices	• Nonliving tissue • Derived from allogenic, xenographic, or synthetic sources • Accelerate healing with minimized scar tissue formation • Promote host cell attachment to topical therapy and migration of keratinocytes, fibroblasts • Controlled degradation of product (collagen products degrade very quickly in comparison) • Viable cells removed to minimize or prevent inflammatory/immunogenic response	• Partial and full-thickness wounds of varying causes • Burn wounds • Traumatic wounds • Surgical wounds	• Applied directly to wound bed using sutures/staples • Acellular matrix hydrated with normal sterile saline • Nonadherent secondary dressing applied to secure acellular matrix into place

(continued on next page)

Table 3
(continued)

Category of Products	Description of Product	Clinical Indications	Instructions for Clinical Use
Placental tissue allografts	• Derived from human amnion/chorion placental membrane or umbilical cord • Deliver exogenous growth factors to the wound bed • Antimicrobial and anti-inflammatory • Collagen rich	• Acute and chronic wounds • Nonhealing wounds of varying causes	• Applied directly to wound bed • Nonadherent contact layer placed on overlying tissue as secondary dressing
Cell-based therapies	• Deliver exogenous growth factors to the wound bed • Viable cells are cultured on different bioabsorbable matrices • Cell-based therapy can be epidermal, dermal, or bilayer therapies • Cells removed from cell-based therapies include hair follicles, sweat glands, blood vessels, and immune cells	• Partial and full-thickness wounds • Chronic nonhealing wounds of differing causes • Burn wounds	• Cell-based therapy applied directly to wound bed and secured with Steri-Strips and nonadherent dressing

granulation tissue, removal of excess wound exudate, improvement in tissue oxygenation, and reduction of bacterial bioburden—all key factors that assist with wound healing.

The direct and indirect physiologic effects of NPWT have had a dramatic positive impact on wound management. The direct effects of NPWT include the use of a semipermeable dressing (enabling a moist/warm environment) and generation of a pressure gradient, which assists in removing exudate from the wound ultimately to the collection canister. NPWT has been shown through numerous studies to be highly successful in assisting with forming granulation tissue over exposed bone, tendon, or orthopedic hardware.[47,48]

From an indirect standpoint, NPWT decreases bacterial bioburden and MMP activity, increases local arterial blood flow, and induces a microstrain on the tissue.[49,50] This microstrain (or cell stretch) increases cellular and growth factor activity, including fibroblasts, vascular endothelial growth factor, and fibroblast growth factor 2.[49] NPWT dressings are often changed every 48 to 72 hours, reducing cross-contamination of the wound and deterring the regrowth of bacterial biofilms on the wound bed.

Applications and indications for the use of NPWT have been expanding, including tunneling wounds or placement over avascular tissue. The optimal subatmospheric pressure setting to maximize blood flow, evacuate exudate, reduce edema, remove bacteria, and facilitate a moist wound environment has been suggested to be 125 mm Hg of pressure alternating between 5 minutes of pressure and 2 minutes of suction.[51] However, further studies have suggested that lower subatmospheric pressure may be just as effective in achieving the desired physiologic effects of NPWT.[52] The clinician also must determine whether to proceed with intermittent or continuous pressure. Studies have suggested that the intermittent setting has been more effective at stimulating angiogenesis and granulation tissue formation.[53] Increased pain and reduced patient acceptance has limited the integration of the intermittent pressure setting into routine clinical practice.

Multiple types of NPWT devices are currently available on the market and have been divided into 4 categories. The first includes the standard NPWT devices that are used in the acute care setting. The second category includes the smaller and more portable devices designed to be used in the outpatient setting. NPWT devices from categories 1 and 2 are battery powered and require frequent charging. The third group includes disposable devices intended to deliver 7 days of NPWT to wounds without charging. The fourth category of NPWT systems has been considered the specialty group, and includes the systems that contain the instillation component as well as NPWT. NPWT with use of instillation and dwell time (NPWTi-d) has also become available in clinical practice, and has further improved the efficiency of granulation tissue formation and reduced bacterial bioburden.[54] NPWTi-d combines the intermittent instillation of a solution topically to the wound, a dwell period permitting the solution to remain on the wound, followed by negative pressure removing the solution. Different solutions have been used with NPWTi-d including normal saline and antiseptics (PHMB); however, there does not appear to be a difference in outcomes regarding a duration of hospital length of stay, number of operative visits, or the proportion of wounds closed at 30 days' duration.[55] Incisional NPWT has also been included in the fourth category of NPWT systems. Incisional NPWT has been shown to assist with the closure of complex/high-risk lower extremity incisions by reducing seroma/hematoma formation,[56] decreasing tensile forces along the incision,[57] and reducing edema[56] (Table 4).

NPWT is a well-tolerated therapy that has become a mainstay in wound care. The clinician, however, should be cognizant of the few contraindications to NPWT

Table 4
Negative pressure wound therapy devices

Descriptions of Products	Benefits	Drawbacks
NPWT devices designed for acute care setting	• Evidence-based results • Support heavy exudative wounds	• Device may be heavy • Charging often required
Portable NPWT devices	• Small in size/lightweight • Designed for use at home	• Not available off-the-shelf • Noise of the device can be bothersome
Disposable NPWT devices	• Light weight • Off-the-shelf availability • Some devices approved for incisional therapy	• Limited pressure levels • Not indicated for moderate to higher exudative wounds
Specialized NPWT • NPWT devices with instillation • Incisional NPWT	• Studies suggest increased proficiency of granulation tissue formation • Reduce wound bioburden • Reduce seroma/hematoma formation	• In-hospital use only (cannot be used in the outpatient setting)

including untreated osteomyelitis or infection, malignancy, exposed vital structures, necrotic tissue within the wound, and nonenteric and unexplored fistulas.

SUMMARY

Following a breach in the skin, wounds should heal in a complex but predictable fashion. When patients fail to progress through these predictable stages of healing, the health care provider must determine the cause of the stalled wound. An appreciation and adherence to the major pillars of wound care including effective offloading strategies, vascular optimization, infection management, and wound-bed preparation are critical to enhanced healing. Adhering to these principles is crucial in expecting successful and timely wound closure. Included with these mainstays of wound care is topical wound and dressing management, which can be defined as manipulating the physiologic environment of the wound bed through the use of dressings, topical therapies, and NPWT to reestablish normal functioning of tissue. There are more than 3000 types of wound-care products on the market today, which can create some confusion with dressing selection. However, appreciation of the needs of the wound along with an understanding of the categories of wound-care products will facilitate this process.

REFERENCES

1. Lazarus GS, Cooper DM, Knighton DR, et al. Definitions and guidelines for assessment of wounds and evaluation of healing. Wound Repair Regen 1994; 2(3):165–70.
2. Gottrup F. A specialized wound-healing center concept: importance of a multidisciplinary department structure and surgical treatment facilities in the treatment of chronic wounds. Am J Surg 2004;187(5A):38S–43S.
3. Crovetti G, Martinelli G, Issi M, et al. Platelet gel for healing cutaneous chronic wounds. Transfus Apher Sci 2004;30(2):145–51.

4. Brem H, Stojadinovic O, Diegelmann RF, et al. Molecular markers in patients with chronic wounds to guide surgical debridement. Mol Med 2007;13(1–2):30–9.

5. Hinman CD, Maibach H. Effect of air exposure and occlusion on experimental human skin wounds. Nature 1963;200:377–8.

6. Hopf HW, Ueno C, Aslam R, et al. Guidelines for the treatment of arterial insufficiency ulcers. Wound Repair Regen 2006;14(6):693–710.

7. Trengove NJ, Stacey MC, MacAuley S, et al. Analysis of the acute and chronic wound environments: the role of proteases and their inhibitors. Wound Repair Regen 1999;7(6):442–52.

8. Dowsett C. Exudate management: a patient-centred approach. J Wound Care 2008;17(6):249–52.

9. Zhang X, Sun D, Jiang G. Comparative efficacy of 9 different dressings in healing diabetic foot ulcer :a bayesian network analysis. J Diabetes 2018. https://doi.org/10.1111/1753-0407.12871.

10. Saco M, Howe N, Nathoo R, et al. Comparing the efficacies of alginate, foam, hydrocolloid, hydrofiber, and hydrogel dressings in the management of diabetic foot ulcers and venous leg ulcers: a systematic review and meta-analysis examining how to dress for success. Dermatol Online J 2016;22(8) [pii: 13030/qt7ph5v17z].

11. Bradley M, Cullum N, Nelson EA, et al. Systematic reviews of wound care management: (2). dressings and topical agents used in the healing of chronic wounds. Health Technol Assess 1999;3(17 Pt 2):1–35.

12. Bouza C, Saz Z, Munoz A, et al. Efficacy of advanced dressings in the treatment of pressure ulcers: a systematic review. J Wound Care 2005;14(5):193–9.

13. Salmeron-Gonzalez E, Garcia-Vilarino E, Ruiz-Cases A, et al. Absorption capacity of wound dressings: a comparative experimental study. Plast Surg Nurs 2018; 38(2):73–5.

14. Kahn S. Highlights from the advanced wound healing stream at the LINK congress. Br J Nurs 2017;26(Sup20):S34–6.

15. Ovington LG. Hanging wet-to-dry dressings out to dry. Home Healthc Nurse 2001;19(8):477–83 [quiz: 484].

16. Sood A, Granick MS, Tomaselli NL. Wound dressings and comparative effectiveness data. Adv Wound Care (New Rochelle) 2014;3(8):511–29.

17. Diehm C, Lawall H. Evaluation of tielle hydropolymer dressings in the management of chronic exuding wounds in primary care. Int Wound J 2005;2(1):26–35.

18. Ohura N, Ichioka S, Nakatsuka T, et al. Evaluating dressing materials for the prevention of shear force in the treatment of pressure ulcers. J Wound Care 2005; 14(9):401–4.

19. Blair SD, Jarvis P, Salmon M, et al. Clinical trial of calcium alginate haemostatic swabs. Br J Surg 1990;77(5):568–70.

20. Jones S, bowler PG, walker M. Antimicrobial activity of silver-containing dressings is influenced by dressing conformability with a wound surface. Wounds 2005;17(9):263–70.

21. Waring MJ, Parsons D. Physico-chemical characterisation of carboxymethylated spun cellulose fibres. Biomaterials 2001;22(9):903–12.

22. Lobmann R, Zemlin C, Motzkau M, et al. Expression of matrix metalloproteinases and growth factors in diabetic foot wounds treated with a protease absorbent dressing. J Diabetes Complications 2006;20(5):329–35.

23. Wainwright DJ. Use of an acellular allograft dermal matrix (AlloDerm) in the management of full-thickness burns. Burns 1995;21(4):243–8.

24. Ulrich D, Smeets R, Unglaub F, et al. Effect of oxidized regenerated cellulose/collagen matrix on proteases in wound exudate of patients with diabetic foot ulcers. J Wound Ostomy Continence Nurs 2011;38(5):522–8.

25. Smeets R, Ulrich D, Unglaub F, et al. Effect of oxidised regenerated cellulose/collagen matrix on proteases in wound exudate of patients with chronic venous ulceration. Int Wound J 2008;5(2):195–203.

26. Spangler D, Rothenburger S, Nguyen K, et al. In vitro antimicrobial activity of oxidized regenerated cellulose against antibiotic-resistant microorganisms. Surg Infect (Larchmt) 2003;4(3):255–62.

27. Gottrup F, Cullen BM, Karlsmark T, et al. Randomized controlled trial on collagen/oxidized regenerated cellulose/silver treatment. Wound Repair Regen 2013;21(2):216–25.

28. Jeschke MG, Sandmann G, Schubert T, et al. Effect of oxidized regenerated cellulose/collagen matrix on dermal and epidermal healing and growth factors in an acute wound. Wound Repair Regen 2005;13(3):324–31.

29. Liden BA, May BC. Clinical outcomes following the use of ovine forestomach matrix (endoform dermal template) to treat chronic wounds. Adv Skin Wound Care 2013;26(4):164–7.

30. Driver V, French M, Cain J, et al. The use of the native collagen dressing on chronic lower extremity wounds, case studies: presented at the symposium on advanced wound care: Presented at the Symposium on Advanced Wound Care. Tampa, FL, 2007.

31. Shah S, Chakravarthy D. A clinical safety and efficacy evaluation on seriously chronic wounds with a native collagen dressing. Puracol Plus clinical report. Internal report, 2007.

32. Wolcott RD, Fletcher J, Phillips PL, et al. Biofilms made easy. Wounds International 2010;1(3). Available at: http://www.woundsinternational.com/.

33. Wolcott RD, Rhoads DD, Bennett ME, et al. Chronic wounds and the medical biofilm paradigm. J Wound Care 2010;19(2):45–6, 48–50, 52–3.

34. Ovington LG. The truth about silver. Ostomy Wound Manage 2004;50(9A Suppl):1S–10S.

35. Fong J, Wood F. Nanocrystalline silver dressings in wound management: a review. Int J Nanomedicine 2006;1(4):441–9.

36. Zou SB, Yoon WY, Han SK, et al. Cytotoxicity of silver dressings on diabetic fibroblasts. Int Wound J 2013;10(3):306–12.

37. Reynolds J. Martindale: the extra pharmacopoeia. 29th edition. London: The Pharmaceutical Press; 1989.

38. Gordon J. Clinical significance of methicillin-sensitive and methicillin-resistant staphylococcus aureus in UK hospitals and the relevance of povidone-iodine in their control. Postgrad Med J 1993;69(Suppl 3):S106–16.

39. Selvaggi G, Monstrey S, Van Landuyt K, et al. The role of iodine in antisepsis and wound management: a reappraisal. Acta Chir Belg 2003;103(3):241–7.

40. Sorensen OE, Cowland JB, Theilgaard-Monch K, et al. Wound healing and expression of antimicrobial peptides/polypeptides in human keratinocytes, a consequence of common growth factors. J Immunol 2003;170(11):5583–9.

41. Butcher M. PHMB: an effective antimicrobial in wound bioburden management. Br J Nurs 2012;21(12):S16. S18-21.

42. Chirife J, Scarmato G, Herszage L. Scientific basis for use of granulated sugar in treatment of infected wounds. Lancet 1982;1(8271):560–1.

43. Topham J. Sugar for wounds. J Tissue Viability 2000;10(3):86–9.

44. Margolis DJ, Kantor J, Berlin JA. Healing of diabetic neuropathic foot ulcers receiving standard treatment. A meta-analysis. Diabetes Care 1999;22(5):692–5.
45. Sheehan P, Jones P, Caselli A, et al. Percent change in wound area of diabetic foot ulcers over a 4-week period is a robust predictor of complete healing in a 12-week prospective trial. Diabetes Care 2003;26(6):1879–82.
46. Heldin CH, Westermark B. Mechanism of action and in vivo role of platelet-derived growth factor. Physiol Rev 1999;79(4):1283–316.
47. DeFranzo AJ, Argenta LC, Marks MW, et al. The use of vacuum-assisted closure therapy for the treatment of lower-extremity wounds with exposed bone. Plast Reconstr Surg 2001;108(5):1184–91.
48. Lee HJ, Kim JW, Oh CW, et al. Negative pressure wound therapy for soft tissue injuries around the foot and ankle. J Orthop Surg Res 2009;4:14.
49. Huang C, Leavitt T, Bayer LR, et al. Effect of negative pressure wound therapy on wound healing. Curr Probl Surg 2014;51(7):301–31.
50. Gough A, Clapperton M, Rolando N, et al. Randomised placebo-controlled trial of granulocyte-colony stimulating factor in diabetic foot infection. Lancet 1997;350(9081):855–9.
51. Venturi ML, Attinger CE, Mesbahi AN, et al. Mechanisms and clinical applications of the vacuum-assisted closure (VAC) device: a review. Am J Clin Dermatol 2005;6(3):185–94.
52. Borgquist O, Gustafsson L, Ingemansson R, et al. Micro- and macromechanical effects on the wound bed of negative pressure wound therapy using gauze and foam. Ann Plast Surg 2010;64(6):789–93.
53. Borgquist O, Ingemansson R, Malmsjo M. The effect of intermittent and variable negative pressure wound therapy on wound edge microvascular blood flow. Ostomy Wound Manage 2010;56(3):60–7.
54. Goss SG, Schwartz JA, Facchin F, et al. Negative pressure wound therapy with instillation (NPWTi) better reduces post-debridement bioburden in chronically infected lower extremity wounds than NPWT alone. J Am Coll Clin Wound Spec 2014;4(4):74–80.
55. Kim PJ, Attinger CE. Reply: comparison of outcomes for normal saline and an antiseptic solution for negative-pressure wound therapy with instillation. Plast Reconstr Surg 2016;137(6):1064e–5e.
56. Pellino G, Sciaudone G, Candilio G, et al. Effects of a new pocket device for negative pressure wound therapy on surgical wounds of patients affected with Crohn's disease: a pilot trial. Surg Innov 2014;21(2):204–12.
57. Wilkes RP, Kilpad DV, Zhao Y, et al. Closed incision management with negative pressure wound therapy (CIM): biomechanics. Surg Innov 2012;19(1):67–75.

Updates on Bioengineered Alternative Tissues

John Miller, DPM[a], Jacob Wynes, DPM, MS, CWS[b],*

KEYWORDS

- Diabetic foot ulcer • Bioengineered tissue • Wound healing • Chronic wounds

KEY POINTS

- The environment and nature of the wounds dictate the appropriate selection of bioengineered tissue alternative.
- With adequate perfusion, routine wound debridement, and mechanical offloading, the use of bioengineered tissue adjuvants increases rates of wound healing.
- Bioengineered tissue alternatives may be categorically divided into cellular and acellular products based on their biochemical properties and function.

THE DIABETIC FOOT ULCER EPIDEMIC

Despite a quarter century of advancements in surgical, technological, and overall categorical management, diabetic foot ulcers (DFUs) continue their burdensome efflorescence on health systems globally.[1] DFUs are often associated with a high risk of limb loss through surgical amputation following infection. DFUs alone are a proven independent predictor of mortality at 10 years,[2,3] and represent an annual cost of treatment in the United States between $9 and 13 billion.[4]

RATIONALE FOR THE USE OF ENGINEERED SKIN SUBSTITUTES

The treatment of DFUs is challenged not only by their multifactorial cause, but also their chronicity and resistance to therapies. Numerous wound care products, offloading devices, and antimicrobial dressings exist for improving DFU healing rates. However, systematic reviews elucidated dismal outcomes with standard-of-care therapies, resulting in only 24% of healed wounds after 12 weeks of care and only 31% after 20 weeks.[5]

Disclosure Statement: The authors have nothing to disclose related to the material presented in this publication.
a Baltimore VA Health System, Rubin Institute for Advanced Orthopedics, 10 North Greene Street, Baltimore, MD 21201, USA; b Department of Orthopaedics, UMMC Limb Preservation Clinic, University of Maryland, University of Maryland School of Medicine, 2200 Kernan Drive, Baltimore, MD 21207, USA
* Corresponding author.
E-mail address: Jwynes@som.umaryland.edu

Clin Podiatr Med Surg 36 (2019) 413–424
https://doi.org/10.1016/j.cpm.2019.02.009
0891-8422/19/© 2019 Elsevier Inc. All rights reserved.

podiatric.theclinics.com

Refractory to these troubling outcomes, bioengineered alternative tissues (BATs) and other advanced treatment modalities were produced to accelerate stalled wound healing and prevent the deleterious complications of prolonged wound healing. Multiple prospective evaluations demonstrate that these treatments have improved healing outcomes for chronic DFUs over that of standard-of-care therapies, without increasing infection or complication rates.[6,7] In 2009 Reyzelman and colleagues[8] in their prospective, randomized, multicenter evaluation of 86 patients with DFUs receiving either standard of care or BAT therapies noted a significant increase in the proportion of healed wounds in the BAT arm (69.6%) compared with the standard care group (46.%) at a 12-week end point. Additionally, the converse was true in that a greater proportion who received standard care remained unhealed (53.8%) versus the study group (30.4%) (**Table 1**).

Sheehan and colleagues[9,10] attempted to establish a marker for predicting when wounds may require advanced wound management versus continued standard of care. By analyzing 203 DFUs and tracking the average wound percentage area reduction at 4- and 12-week intervals, Sheehan noted that the percent improvement in DFUs during the first 4 weeks of therapy is a strong predictor of the wound's

Table 1
Brief overview of the composition and function of selected BATs reviewed in this article

Product Name	Components	Function
Cellular (dermoinductive) products		
Theraskin	Cryopreserved split-thickness cadaveric skin allograft	Living fibroblasts and keratinocytes produce growth factors, cytokines, and collagen
Dermagraft	Allogeneic fetal fibroblasts seeded onto a polyglactin matrix	Fibroblasts secrete growth factors and ECM to stimulate autologous epithelization
Apligraf	Neonatal foreskin with bovine collagen	Produces growth factors and matrix proteins to stimulate proliferation and differentiation
Epifix	Bilayer amniotic and chorion membrane	Rich in ECM, producing numerous proteins and growth factors to accelerate wound regeneration
Hyalomatrix	Hyaluronic acid matrix	Component of ECM promotes fibroblast proliferation and angiogenesis
Acellular (dermoconductive) products		
Oasis	Porcine small intestine submucosa	Acellular scaffold containing growth factors and collagen
Integra	Bovine collagen and chondroitin-6-sulfate with silicone covering	Acts as a vascular scaffold facilitating vascular ingrowth and graft population with host fibroblasts
Acell	Porcine bladder matrix	Scaffold of collagens, GAGs, and growth factors similar to human tissue
Primatrix	Dermal collagen scaffold from bovine forestomach	Acellular scaffold with abundant type III collagen

Abbreviations: ECM, extracellular matrix; GAG, glycosaminoglycans.

likelihood to be healed at 12 weeks. Therefore, wounds that do not demonstrate significant improvement in their initial 4 weeks of improvement likely best benefit by use of BATs.

To understand the effectiveness of biochemically engineered tissue constructs, one must first remember the stages of homeostasis wound healing.

LIMITATIONS TO THE USE OF ADVANCED TISSUES ADJUVANTS

Regardless of the efficacy of any advanced skin substitute product, fundamentals of wound healing remain paramount to ensuring DFU resolution. In the presence of profound tissue ischemia or hypoxia, uncontrolled infection, or unmitigated biomechanical imbalance, wound healing is likely not possible regardless of the advanced therapy used. Additionally, routine wound care including regular debridement, irrigation, and regular dressing changes are necessary for the success of any advanced treatment modality.[11]

It cannot be emphasized enough, without adequate tissue perfusion wounds cannot be expected to heal regardless of treatment modality. In the setting of macroangiopathy atherosclerotic obstructive disease is likely present to large vessels because of chronic low-density lipoprotein oxidation and plaque deposition. In the setting of tissue loss with clinically altered vascular perfusion, at minimum a diagnostic angiogram by vascular surgery is warranted. Microangiopathy may also be contributing to local tissue hypoxia. Decreased nitric oxide and prostaglandin secretion, smooth muscle relaxation, and arteriovenous shunting secondary to autonomic neuropathy all contribute to decreased vasodilation and membrane permeability following tissue damage. Cumulatively this leads to a sluggish vascular response and inhibits ability of diffusion at the capillary level.

In addition to tissue hypoxia, a host of local factors exist to inhibit homeostatic wound healing.[12–14] Chronic inflammation prolongs the chemotaxis of cytokines and destructive matrix metalloproteinases leading to an "inflammatory soup" and a seemingly stalled inflammatory phase of healing. Moisture imbalances from chronic exudate drainage desiccated tissue structure. So-called "senescent" fibroblasts become inhibited by the oxidative stressors found in chronic wounds, ultimately receiving enough exposure to free oxygen radicals to trigger cellular apoptosis.[15–17]

BIOENGINEERED ALTERNATIVE TISSUES

In 2007 Steinberg and colleagues[18] introduced the language dermoinductive and dermoconductive as both a descriptive and functional classification separating orthobiologic graft materials. The authors separated materials into acellular (dermoconductive) and cellular (dermoinductive) to elucidate the difference between products working as a functional scaffold in comparison with those containing actual living cells that contribute to wound maturation through exogenous methods.

As a generalization, acellular products tend to be more porous and to allow binding and integration into the host substrate. Acellular products rely on the modulation of host DNA to secrete various growth factors including collagen, hyaluronic acid (HA), and fibronectin.

Acellular scaffold matrices function by allowing free-flowing wound exudate containing epithelial cells, fibroblasts, and vascular endothelial cells to migrate into graft scaffold to bind and proliferate. As an added benefit, harmful free metalloproteinases also bind to graft collagen, rebalancing the ratio of proteases and growth factors to chronic wounds. Examples of acellular or dermoconductive products include bilayer xenografts or porcine intestinal mucosa.[19]

Most cellular or dermoinductive products are made of fibroblasts and keratinocytes within collagen or a polyglactin scaffold. These cells are essential for the induction of new granulation tissue and epithelial "neodermis." Because of their living cellular composition cellular tissues are more akin to split-thickness skin grafts, than traditional scaffold matrices.[20] Classic examples of cellular matrices include Apligraf (Organogenesis, Canton, MA), Dermagraft (Organogenesis), and EpiFix (Mimedx group Inc, Marietta, GA).

Currently greater than 60 "skin substitute" BAT products are approved by Medicare for use in wound care. Despite such plethora of options, few products have undergone randomized controlled trials (RCTs), with a fraction of products completing investigation worthy of Food and Drug Administration (FDA) approval.[21] Investigators Lev-Tov and colleagues[22] are conducting a prospective, blinded RCT evaluating the cost effectiveness between cellular and acellular wound matrix devices in DFU. Further work in this area will continue to add valuable data to support the best rationalization of cost expenditures without compromising patient outcomes. Similar studies may also provide additional understanding regarding the indications and contraindications for preferring one BAT over another.

CELLULAR (DERMOINDUCTIVE) PRODUCTS
EpiFix

Epifix (Mimedx Group Inc) is a bilayer amniotic allograft membrane consisting of an amnion and chorion layer. This bioengineered alternative is rich in extracellular membrane (ECM) containing collagen types I, III, IV, V, and VII, and proteins, fibronectin, proteoglycans, and glycosaminoglycans (GAGs). Exogenous Epifix also produces growth factors, such as epidermal growth factor, transforming growth factor, fibroblast growth factor, and platelet-derived growth factor, to accelerate wound regeneration.[23,24]

Garoufalis and colleagues[25] investigated the use of Epifix in patients with diabetic wounds who had not met greater than 50% healing after 4 weeks of standard treatment. Wound type origins were classified as 35% DFU, 25% venous leg ulceration (VLU), 20% surgical, 14% pressure, 6% ischemic, and 2% traumatic. A total of 91% of wounds were documented to reach complete healing following 5.1 ± 4.2 applications of Epifix (n = 117 with 101 completing treatment).

Multiple additional authors have published impressive outcomes for the treatment of lower extremity wounds using Epifix. Bianchi and colleagues[26] demonstrated 60% wound closure rate of VLUs at 12 weeks following serial application. Other authors have published DFU healing rates ranging from 80% to 92% at 6 weeks,[24,27] and 87.5% at average of 9 weeks.[28]

Amniotic tissues may also inhibit the accumulation of biofilms. Recent evidence from Mao and colleagues[29] demonstrate the ability of cryopreserved viable amniotic or umbilical tissues to initiate antibacterial activity against multiple pathogens. Specifically, the formation of *Pseudomonas aeruginosa* and *Staphylococcus aureus* was reduced 97% and 72%, respectively, compared with the biofilm formation on the control tissues following their application.

Hyalomatrix/Hyaff

HA (Medline, Northfield IL) matrices area nonsulfated GAG consisting of a highly polymerized chain of N-acetylglucosamine and glucuronic acid. HA is a major component of the ECM throughout human tissues and is primarily produced following fibroblast activation during the initial inflammatory cascade of the wound healing cycle. Because of its integration into the ECM, HA participates in a variety of cell surface receptor functions. Exogenous HA application is demonstrated to promote fibroblast proliferation and angiogenesis[30] while also maintaining antioxidative and anti-inflammatory properties.[31]

Deep wounds present a unique difficulty for accelerated healing, particularly when containing exposed tendinous or osseous structures. Replacement of lost ECM in deep wounds is beneficial to the development of quality granulation tissue and to expedite healing. Simman and colleagues[32] also demonstrated the use of HA for the coverage of exposed tendon in 12 patients with large soft tissue defects. HA matrices have also been implicated in adipogenesis for the repair of large soft tissue defects.

Multiple versions of HA tissue therapy exist, all with the goal of replacing lost ECM and encouraging the production of a "neodermis." Hyaff (Medline) is an esterified form of HA combining stable benzyl esters of HA with a second layer of protective, semipermeable silicone membrane that may be removed for further grafting as indicated.

Apligraf

Apligraf (Organogenesis) was the first commercially available engineered biologic tissue entering the market in 1998. Apligraf is FDA approved for the treatment of DFU and consists of a bilayer tissue of one-part neonatal foreskin and a second derived from bovine collagen. This combination resembles that of epidermis and dermis and stimulates cellular proliferation by producing growth factors and matrix proteins. Early primary indications for the use of Apligraf were relegated to venous leg ulcers; however, 2 years following additional FDA approval, Apligraf was approved for use in neuropathic diabetic wounds greater than 3 weeks of duration.[33]

Investigations conducted by Veves and colleagues[34] demonstrated its effectiveness in nonischemic DFU. In 2001 Veves conducted a prospective RCT using Apligraf versus saline-moistened gauze in 208 patients with diabetes with noninfected, nonischemic wounds. A total of 56% of the Apligraf group achieved healing, compared with 38% in the moistened-saline gauze control. Additionally, time to healing in the trial group was 65 days compared with 90 days in the control group.

Apligraf is limited by its need for repeat applications, and functionally by a shelf-life of 10 days. However, when comparing the reduction in cost from expedited wound healing with extended visitations and hospitalizations Apligraf and other cellular adjuvants may be considered cost-effective alternatives to tissue healing.[35]

Dermagraft

Dermagraft (Organogenesis) is a cell-based dermal substitute composed of human fibroblasts derived from a single neonatal foreskin donor source, which have been seeded onto a bioabsorbable polyglactin matrix. When applied to bleeding tissue the fibroblasts and secret ECM accelerate tissue granulation and re-epithelization. The cellular scaffold functions to stimulate autologous host tissue response rather than permanent graft incorporation.[36]

Multiple large retrospective studies have evaluated the effectiveness of Dermagraft against standard saline-moist dressings. Gentzkow and colleagues[37] established weekly applications of a single sheet of Dermagraft was superior to weekly applications of dual sheets and single sheet applications in 2 weeks cycles. Of the three study arms examined, 50% of patients receiving the single, weekly application completed 100% wound closure at 8 weeks.

In 2003 Marston and colleagues[38] published an article outlining the efficacy and safety of Dermagraft in comparison with conventional wound therapy, demonstrating a 30% healing of recalcitrant diabetic wounds over a 12-week period. This was nearly double the 18.3% healing rate in the control group of standard care. Adverse effects were equivalent between the two arms. Marston and colleagues[38] noted that Dermagraft must be used as an adjunct therapy in addition to standard wound care practices stating that the application of a skin substitute without adhering to the standard wound care practices would likely not result in improved rates of healing.

Limitations to Dermagraft include its required storage at −75°C; need for multiple applications; and presence of bovine proteins and storage materials, which have resulted in hypersensitivity reactions in a small number of patients. However, many of these disadvantages are offset by its ease of handling, and lack of foreign body immune response.

Theraskin

Theraskin (Soluble Systems, Newport News, VA) is a cryopreserved allograft harvested from human cadaveric skin. Being allograft material, Theraskin is reportedly able to deliver a wider complex of growth factors and cytokines as compared with other acellular products.[39] Landsman and colleagues[40] analyzed the cellular makeup of Theraskin and determined the amounts of type I and III collagen were present in equivalent quantity and ratio as in unprocessed split-thickness skin. Additionally, similar quantities of vascular endothelial growth factor, insulin-like growth factor-1, fibroblast growth factor-2, and transforming growth factor B1 were present in the cadaveric tissue as compared with fresh human skin.

In 2018 a prospective, blinded, head-to-head RCT comparing Apligraf with Theraskin outcomes in VLUs was published by Towler and colleagues.[41] Although Theraskin and Apligraf cohorts demonstrated increased healing rates at 12 weeks (93.3% and 75.0%, respectively) and 20 weeks (93.3% and 83.3%, respectively), the authors noted a 42.2% decrease in cost when using the same size Theraskin graft as compared with Apligraf.[41]

ACELLULAR (DERMOCONDUCTIVE) PRODUCTS
Oasis

Oasis (Smith and Nephew, Andover, MA) is a porcine xenograft derived from the small intestinal submucosa of swine. Life other acellular graft products Oasis does not contain living cells. However, it has the components of dermal ECM, such as collagen, elastin, proteoglycans, glycoproteins, and GAG, which function as a scaffold to absorb bioactive molecules and cytokines.[42] Because of its preparation, Oasis is benefitted by a long shelf-life, rapid application, and lower cost than other BATs and as a result is often used a control treatment when evaluating the outcomes of new BAT products.

In 2016 published Oasis outcomes were evaluated in a Cochrane systematic review by Santema and colleagues[43] in comparison with similar trials using cellular based BATs. This review reinforced the previous findings by Gilligan and coworkers[44] and Landsman and coworkers[45] that treatment costs using cellular based BATs are approximately 50% greater than when using Oasis alone.

Integra

Originally designed for use in burn injuries, Integra (Integra LifeSciences, Plainsboro, NJ) is now a commonly used wound adjuvant composed of adult bovine cross-linked type-1 tendon collagen and shark chondroitin-6-sulfate covered with a second, outer layer of protective silicone padding. Integra Bilayer wound matrix provides a scaffold matrix for cellular migration and proliferation similar to other acellular BATs while minimizing the host inflammatory response **(Fig. 1)**.[46]

Integra is a robust substrate for application over exposed tendon and bone.[47,48] Clerici and colleagues[48] evaluated 30 patients with DFUs involving exposed tendon or bone who were treated with initial debridement and Integra application. During treatment 16/30 patients received revascularization by surgical intervention and complete wound healing was noted in 86.7% of patients without major complication noted. Integra is continuously used as a part of a surgically staged wound management, typically applied after wound debridement to potentiate repair in large soft tissue defects before application of split-thickness graft or other cellular matrix for epithelization.[49] Iorio and colleagues[50] demonstrated functional salvage of wound defects in high-risk patients equivalent to that of a lower risk population with similar wounds following the use of Integra.

Acell

Acell (Acell Inc, Columbia, MD) is among a newer generation of a urinary porcine bladder matrix in multiple formulations including a micronized powder, and single or multilayer sheets, and a multilaminate vacuum-pressed sheet of varying thickness. The urinary porcine bladder is a tissue-derived, non-cross-linked scaffold whose biocomposition includes collagens, GAG, and growth factors in similar concentration to that of human dermis.[51]

In 2004 Demling and colleagues[52] conducted a prospective trial for VLUs comparing Acell xenograft against standard treatment. At 12 weeks the xenograft arm noted 71% healing rate as compared with 46% receiving standard treatment. Surprisingly, an additional trial evaluating the efficacy of Acell in VLUs demonstrated a 55% healing rate even without use of compression therapy.[53] In a prospective outcome's comparison of HA versus Acell xenograft, Romanelli and colleagues[54] demonstrated 82% wound healing at 16 weeks.

Additionally, in a comparative analysis of skin substitutes performed by Martinson and Martinson[55] in 2016 using Medicare claims data of more than 13,000 episodes,

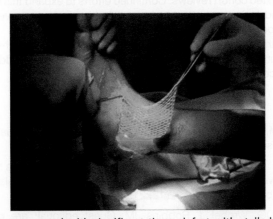

Fig. 1. The patient presented with significant tissue defect with stalled wound improvement. Use of acellular BAT promoted the rapid development of healthy, granular tissue through reactivation of host healing response. A meshed split-thickness skin graft is applied to expedite wound healing and reduce risk of wound infection.

porcine bladder was determined to be equivalent and noninferior to porcine intestinal mucosa. In the review both modalities of porcine-derived grafts reduced lengths of DFU episodes when compared with standard-of-care treatments.

The authors note the powder tends to integrate into the host wound the fastest, with the increasing thickness of sheets taking up to multiple weeks to fully incorporate.

Primatrix

Primatrix (Integra LifeSciences) is a dermal collagen scaffold processed from dermis, specifically composed of layers of propria-submucosa from fetal bovine forestomach. It is therefore an acellular matrix and rich in type III collagen.[56]

Kavros and colleagues[56] conducted a multicenter, prospective RCT comparing chronic DFU outcomes with twice weekly applications of Primatrix. Forty-six patients completed the study term and documented an average wound area reduction of 71.4%, with 76% of wounds reaching complete healing by 12 weeks. These results matched Liden and May[57] who in a review of 19 patients with chronic wounds demonstrated 50% healing at 12 weeks.

SUMMARY

BATs occupy a niche space in the treatment ladder for DFUs. The failure of standard therapy, large soft tissue defects, and rapid development of granular wound bed before application of split-thickness skin grafts or other cellular skin substitute, is a desirable application for this treatment modality. However, because of their higher costs, many hospital systems may limit the available products or refuse to use them altogether.

Without the fundamental basics of wound care including maximizing tissue perfusion, offloading, routine debridement, and treatment of local infection, limited to no success with any advanced wound care modality should be expected. Biologics do not work in the presence of significant mechanical deformity, profound tissue ischemia/hypoxia, and uncontrolled infection.

Despite the quantity of multicenter, blinded, prospective reviews significantly increasing over the past 10 years, much of the remaining literature falls into either case series or limited cohort reviews. Continued efforts to expand this area of research will not only lead to better patient outcomes but may also uncover new areas of research and production.

In conclusion the use of BATs will likely only continue to dominate the outpatient and perioperative management of chronic, recalcitrant wounds as new additional products continue to cut costs and improve wound healing expectations.

REFERENCES

1. Boulton AJM, Vileikyte L, Ragnarson-Tennvall G, et al. The global burden of diabetic foot disease. Lancet 2005;366(9498):1719–24.

2. Iversen MM, Tell GS, Riise T, et al. History of foot ulcer increases mortality among individuals with diabetes: ten-year follow-up of the Nord-Trøndelag Health Study, Norway. Diabetes Care 2009;32(12):2193–9.

3. Armstrong DG, Wrobel J, Robbins JM. Guest editorial: are diabetes-related wounds and amputations worse than cancer? Int Wound J 2007;4(4):286–7.

4. Rice JB, Desai U, Cummings AKG, et al. Burden of diabetic foot ulcers for Medicare and private insurers. Diabetes Care 2014;37(3):651–8.

5. Margolis DJ, Kantor J, Berlin JA. Healing of diabetic neuropathic foot ulcers receiving standard treatment. A meta-analysis. Diabetes Care 1999;22(5): 692–5. Available at: https://www.ncbi.nlm.nih.gov/pubmed/10332667.

6. Winters CL, Brigido SA, Liden BA, et al. A multicenter study involving the use of a human acellular dermal regenerative tissue matrix for the treatment of diabetic lower extremity wounds. Adv Skin Wound Care 2008;21(8):375–81.

7. Snyder RJ, Hanft JR. Diabetic foot ulcers—effects on quality of life, costs, and mortality and the role of standard wound care and advanced-care therapies in healing: a review. Ostomy Wound Manage 2009;55(11):28. Available at: https://pdfs.semanticscholar.org/8ede/209936ed858cf280876c20ded0cee45d36aa.pdf.

8. Reyzelman A, Crews RT, Moore JC, et al. Clinical effectiveness of an acellular dermal regenerative tissue matrix compared to standard wound management in healing diabetic foot ulcers: a prospective, randomised, multicentre study. Int Wound J 2009;6(3):196–208.

9. Sheehan P, Jones P, Caselli A, et al. Percent change in wound area of diabetic foot ulcers over a 4-week period is a robust predictor of complete healing in a 12-week prospective trial. Diabetes Care 2003;26(6):1879–82. Available at: https://www.ncbi.nlm.nih.gov/pubmed/12766127.

10. Singer AJ, Clark RA. Cutaneous wound healing. N Engl J Med 1999;341(10): 738–46.

11. Kim PJ, Steinberg JS. Wound care: biofilm and its impact on the latest treatment modalities for ulcerations of the diabetic foot. Semin Vasc Surg 2012;25(2):70–4.

12. Schultz GS, Sibbald RG, Falanga V, et al. Wound bed preparation: a systematic approach to wound management. Wound Repair Regen 2003;11(Suppl 1): S1–28. Available at: https://www.ncbi.nlm.nih.gov/pubmed/12654015.

13. Wolcott RD, Rhoads DD, Dowd SE. Biofilms and chronic wound inflammation. J Wound Care 2008;17(8):333–41.

14. Cook H, Davies KJ, Harding KG, et al. Defective extracellular matrix reorganization by chronic wound fibroblasts is associated with alterations in TIMP-1, TIMP-2, and MMP-2 activity. J Invest Dermatol 2000;115(2):225–33.

15. Wlaschek M, Scharffetter-Kochanek K. Oxidative stress in chronic venous leg ulcers. Wound Repair Regen 2005;13(5):452–61.

16. Wall IB, Moseley R, Baird DM, et al. Fibroblast dysfunction is a key factor in the non-healing of chronic venous leg ulcers. J Invest Dermatol 2008;128(10): 2526–40.

17. Sorrell JM, Baber MA, Caplan AI. Human dermal fibroblast subpopulations; differential interactions with vascular endothelial cells in coculture: nonsoluble factors in the extracellular matrix influence interactions. Wound Repair Regen 2008; 16(2):300–9.

18. Steinberg JS, Werber B, Kim PJ. Bioengineered alternative tissues for the surgical management of diabetic foot ulceration. In: Zgonis T, editor. Surgical reconstruction of the diabetic foot and ankle. Philadelphia: Lippincott, Williams & Wilkins; 2009. p. 105–9. Available at: https://books.google.com/books?hl=en&lr=&id=LJIgAh0DESEC&oi=fnd&pg=PA100&dq=steinberg+bioengineered+alternative+tissue+2009&ots=0VK_VKfhDy&sig=GtTjC0akH58XraCIA3y4VBxdXZE.

19. Bonadio J, Smiley E, Patil P, et al. Localized, direct plasmid gene delivery in vivo: prolonged therapy results in reproducible tissue regeneration. Nat Med 1999; 5(7):753–9.

20. Luu YK, Kim K, Hsiao BS, et al. Development of a nanostructured DNA delivery scaffold via electrospinning of PLGA and PLA-PEG block copolymers. J Control Release 2003;89(2):341–53. Available at: https://www.ncbi.nlm.nih.gov/pubmed/12711456.

21. Kirsner RS, Sabolinski ML, Parsons NB, et al. Comparative effectiveness of a bio-engineered living cellular construct vs. a dehydrated human amniotic membrane allograft for the treatment of diabetic foot ulcers in a real world setting. Wound Repair Regen 2015;23(5):737–44. Available at: https://onlinelibrary.wiley.com/doi/abs/10.1111/wrr.12332.

22. Lev-Tov H, Li C-S, Dahle S, et al. Cellular versus acellular matrix devices in treatment of diabetic foot ulcers: study protocol for a comparative efficacy randomized controlled trial. Trials 2013;14:8.

23. Koob TJ, Lim JJ, Massee M, et al. Properties of dehydrated human amnion/chorion composite grafts: implications for wound repair and soft tissue regeneration. J Biomed Mater Res B Appl Biomater 2014;102(6):1353–62.

24. Zelen CM, Serena TE, Denoziere G, et al. A prospective randomised comparative parallel study of amniotic membrane wound graft in the management of diabetic foot ulcers. Int Wound J 2013;10(5):502–7.

25. Garoufalis M, Nagesh D, Sanchez PJ, et al. Use of dehydrated human amnion/chorion membrane allografts in more than 100 patients with six major types of refractory nonhealing wounds. J Am Podiatr Med Assoc 2018;108(2):84–9.

26. Bianchi C, Cazzell S, Vayser D, et al. A multicentre randomised controlled trial evaluating the efficacy of dehydrated human amnion/chorion membrane (EpiFix) allograft for the treatment of venous leg ulcers. Int Wound J 2018;15(1):114–22.

27. Couture M. A single-center, retrospective study of cryopreserved umbilical cord for wound healing in patients suffering from chronic wounds of the foot and ankle. Wounds 2016;28(7):217–25. Available at: https://www.ncbi.nlm.nih.gov/pubmed/27428716.

28. Raphael A. A single-centre, retrospective study of cryopreserved umbilical cord/amniotic membrane tissue for the treatment of diabetic foot ulcers. J Wound Care 2016;25(Sup7):S10–7.

29. Mao Y, Singh-Varma A, Hoffman T, et al. The effect of cryopreserved human placental tissues on biofilm formation of wound-associated pathogens. J Funct Biomater 2018;9(1). https://doi.org/10.3390/jfb9010003.

30. Prosdocimi M, Bevilacqua C. Exogenous hyaluronic acid and wound healing: an updated vision. Panminerva Med 2012;54(2):129–35. Available at: https://www.ncbi.nlm.nih.gov/pubmed/22525567.

31. Litwiniuk M, Krejner A, Speyrer MS, et al. Hyaluronic acid in inflammation and tissue regeneration. Wounds 2016;28(3):78–88. Available at: https://www.ncbi.nlm.nih.gov/pubmed/26978861.

32. Simman R, Mari W, Younes S, et al. Use of hyaluronic acid-based biological bilaminar matrix in wound bed preparation: a case series. Eplasty 2018;18:e17. Available at: https://www.ncbi.nlm.nih.gov/pubmed/29765486.

33. Metcalfe AD, Ferguson MWJ. Tissue engineering of replacement skin: the crossroads of biomaterials, wound healing, embryonic development, stem cells and regeneration. J R Soc Interface 2007;4(14):413–37.

34. Veves A, Falanga V, Armstrong DG, et al, Apligraf Diabetic Foot Ulcer Study. Graftskin, a human skin equivalent, is effective in the management of noninfected neuropathic diabetic foot ulcers: a prospective randomized multicenter clinical trial. Diabetes Care 2001;24(2):290–5. Available at: https://www.ncbi.nlm.nih.gov/pubmed/11213881.

35. Redekop WK, McDonnell J, Verboom P, et al. The cost effectiveness of Apligraf treatment of diabetic foot ulcers. Pharmacoeconomics 2003;21(16): 1171–83.
36. Felder JM 3rd, Goyal SS, Attinger CE. A systematic review of skin substitutes for foot ulcers. Plast Reconstr Surg 2012;130(1):145–64.
37. Gentzkow GD, Iwasaki SD, Hershon KS, et al. Use of Dermagraft, a cultured human dermis, to treat diabetic foot ulcers. Diabetes Care 1996;19(4):350–4. Available at: https://www.ncbi.nlm.nih.gov/pubmed/8729158.
38. Marston WA, Hanft J, Norwood P, et al, Dermagraft Diabetic Foot Ulcer Study Group. The efficacy and safety of Dermagraft in improving the healing of chronic diabetic foot ulcers: results of a prospective randomized trial. Diabetes Care 2003;26(6):1701–5.
39. Cook EA, Cook JJ, Badri H, et al. Bioengineered alternative tissues. Clin Podiatr Med Surg 2014;31(1):89–101.
40. Landsman A, Rosines E, Houck A, et al. Characterization of a cryopreserved split-thickness human skin allograft–TheraSkin. Adv Skin Wound Care 2016; 29(9):399.
41. Towler MA, Rush EW, Richardson MK, et al. Randomized, prospective, blinded-enrollment, head-to-head venous leg ulcer healing trial comparing living, bioengineered skin graft substitute (Apligraf) with living, cryopreserved, human skin allograft (TheraSkin). Clin Podiatr Med Surg 2018;35(3):357–65.
42. Garwood CS, Steinberg JS, Kim PJ. Bioengineered alternative tissues in diabetic wound healing. Clin Podiatr Med Surg 2015;32(1):121–33.
43. Santema TBK, Poyck PPC, Ubbink DT. Systematic review and meta-analysis of skin substitutes in the treatment of diabetic foot ulcers: highlights of a Cochrane systematic review. Wound Repair Regen 2016;24(4):737–44. Available at: https://onlinelibrary.wiley.com/doi/abs/10.1111/wrr.12434.
44. Gilligan AM, Waycaster CR, Landsman AL. Wound closure in patients with DFU: a cost-effectiveness analysis of two cellular/tissue-derived products. J Wound Care 2015;24(3):149–56.
45. Landsman A, Roukis TS, DeFronzo DJ, et al. Living cells or collagen matrix: which is more beneficial in the treatment of diabetic foot ulcers? Wounds 2008;20(5): 111–6. Available at: https://www.ncbi.nlm.nih.gov/pubmed/25942411.
46. Kim PJ, Attinger CE, Steinberg JS, et al. Integra bilayer wound matrix application for complex lower extremity soft tissue reconstruction. Surg Technol Int 2014;24: 65–73. Available at: https://www.ncbi.nlm.nih.gov/pubmed/24700214.
47. Silverstein G. Dermal regeneration template in the surgical management of diabetic foot ulcers: a series of five cases. J Foot Ankle Surg 2006;45(1): 28–33.
48. Clerici G, Caminiti M, Curci V, et al. The use of a dermal substitute (integra) to preserve maximal foot length in a diabetic foot wound with bone and tendon exposure following urgent surgical debridement for an acute infection. Int J Low Extrem Wounds 2009;8(4):209–12.
49. Scalise A, Torresetti M, Grassetti L, et al. Acellular dermal matrix and skin grafts: a long-lasting alternative for weightbearing zone reconstruction after degloving trauma of the foot. Musculoskelet Regen 2015;2:e1048. Available at: https://pdfs.semanticscholar.org/02f0/15ec8ebe2e46fd321f8f092c79db1542e2e7.pdf.
50. Iorio ML, Goldstein J, Adams M, et al. Functional limb salvage in the diabetic patient: the use of a collagen bilayer matrix and risk factors for amputation. Plast Reconstr Surg 2011;127(1):260–7.

51. Geiger SE, Deigni OA, Watson JT, et al. Management of open distal lower extremity wounds with exposed tendons using porcine urinary bladder matrix. Wounds 2016;28(9):306–16. Available at: https://www.ncbi.nlm.nih.gov/pubmed/27701126.

52. Demling RH, Niezgoda JA, Haraway GD, et al. Small intestinal submucosa wound matrix and full-thickness venous ulcers: preliminary results. Wounds 2004;16(1): 18–22. Available at: https://www.researchgate.net/profile/Jeffrey_Niezgoda/publication/237618625_Small_Intestinal_Submucosa_Wound_Matrix_and_Full-thic kness_Venous_Ulcers_Preliminary_Results/links/543bd8d40cf2d6698be33f94.pdf.

53. Mostow EN, Haraway GD, Dalsing M, et al, OASIS Venus Ulcer Study Group. Effectiveness of an extracellular matrix graft (OASIS Wound Matrix) in the treatment of chronic leg ulcers: a randomized clinical trial. J Vasc Surg 2005;41(5): 837–43.

54. Romanelli M, Dini V, Bertone M, et al. OASIS wound matrix versus Hyaloskin in the treatment of difficult-to-heal wounds of mixed arterial/venous aetiology. Int Wound J 2007;4(1):3–7. Available at: https://onlinelibrary.wiley.com/doi/abs/10.1111/j.1742-481X.2007.00300.x.

55. Martinson M, Martinson N. A comparative analysis of skin substitutes used in the management of diabetic foot ulcers. J Wound Care 2016;25(Sup10):S8–17.

56. Kavros SJ, Dutra T, Gonzalez-Cruz R, et al. The use of PriMatrix, a fetal bovine acellular dermal matrix, in healing chronic diabetic foot ulcers: a prospective multicenter study. Adv Skin Wound Care 2014;27(8):356–62.

57. Liden BA, May BCH. Clinical outcomes following the use of ovine forestomach matrix (Endoform dermal template) to treat chronic wounds. Adv Skin Wound Care 2013;26(4):164–7.

Soft Tissue Reconstruction with Diabetic Foot Tissue Loss

Todd A. Hasenstein, DPM[a], Timothy Greene, DPM[a],
Jennifer C. Van, DPM[b], Andrew J. Meyr, DPM[b],*

KEYWORDS

- Excisional debridement • Gangrene • Infection • Partial foot amputation
- Soft tissue reconstruction • Fillet of toe • Spaghetti • Reconstructive elevator

KEY POINTS

- Diabetic foot tissue loss often occurs in predictable anatomic patterns. Knowledge of these patterns can assist physicians in minimizing the initial tissue loss associated with infection, as well as guide soft tissue reconstruction.
- The forefoot is the anatomic area most commonly involved in diabetic foot disease. A systematic approach to its evaluation and management might prevent more proximal amputation.
- The midfoot, rearfoot, and ankle might be more amenable to soft tissue reconstruction using the principles as outlined by the reconstructive ladder.

Although it is likely that substantial contemporary advances have been made in the treatment of diabetic foot disease with respect to patient education, preventative measures, early intervention, and prophylactic procedures, it is still unfortunately just as likely that most surgical interventions for this condition are reactionary in nature.[1–8] Patients still frequently primarily present to outpatient physician offices and emergency departments with acute infectious events and resultant tissue necrosis. By definition, the appropriate surgical intervention for this presentation results in a soft tissue deficit, often with partial foot amputation, through the excisional debridement of pathologic tissue. The science and art of minimizing this initial soft tissue loss, along with subsequent reconstruction of the defect, forms the focus of this article.

Disclosure Statement: The authors have nothing to disclose.
[a] Temple University Hospital Podiatric Surgical Residency Program, 8th at Race Street, Philadelphia, PA 19107, USA; [b] Department of Surgery, Temple University School of Podiatric Medicine, 8th at Race Street, Philadelphia, PA 19107, USA
* Corresponding author.
E-mail address: ajmeyr@gmail.com

One potential advantage that surgeons have in treating this condition is that the tissue loss that occurs secondary to infection presents in relatively predictable ways. In fact, the pathway to tissue loss is usually simple: chronic pressure over osseous prominences leads to ulceration, which represents a portal for infection and subsequent tissue necrosis. Chronic pressure in the lower extremity further generally occurs in expected anatomic locations for the forefoot, midfoot, and rearfoot.

FOREFOOT PATHOANATOMY, SURGICAL RESECTION, AND SOFT TISSUE RECONSTRUCTION

The most frequent location for the occurrence of a diabetic foot ulceration is the forefoot.[9–11] This is likely because of the unusual shape of the digits with increased surface area and intimate bone-on-bone contact, the increased likelihood of the presence of deformity, and the high percentage of the tissue that is bone as opposed to soft tissue when considering volume. Consider the cross-sectional anatomy of a digit, for example, and compare the ratio of bone/soft tissue of these appendages with more proximal areas of the foot (**Fig. 1**). In other words, there is relatively more bone and less soft tissue in the distal forefoot compared with other anatomic areas. Therefore, an ulceration and infection must physically penetrate through less tissue to reach deep anatomic structures and tissue planes. Specifically within the forefoot, the most common locations for initial ulceration are the distal tip of the digit, the dorsal aspect of the proximal interphalangeal joint, and plantarly under the metatarsal heads. If infection occurs in one of these areas, the subsequent patterns of tissue destruction might be anticipated with application of anatomic knowledge.

Distal Digital Tip: Pathoanatomy

These ulcerations occur most frequently as a result of ill-fitting shoegear or sagittal plane digital deformity resulting in increased load on the tip of the toe instead of the plantar pulp (**Fig. 2**). Although this might certainly occur in a foot without a history of diabetic foot disease, it is also likely to occur in a foot that has previously undergone partial amputation as the musculoskeletal biomechanical balances are altered.[12] The resultant progressive tissue loss occurs primarily in a localized manner within the fat pad on the plantar pulp. A probe might be expected to course directly deep to the tuft of the distal phalanx and plantarly underneath the distal phalanx near the insertion of the long flexor tendon. However, this is often also accompanied by tissue loss

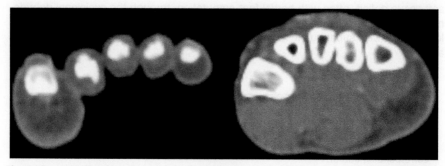

Fig. 1. Cross-sectional anatomy of the foot. Note how the digits have a relatively high ratio of bone to soft tissue, whereas more proximal areas of the foot have relatively more soft tissue. Therefore, ulcerations and infections involving the digits have physically less tissue to penetrate before there is involvement of bone and other deep tissue structures.

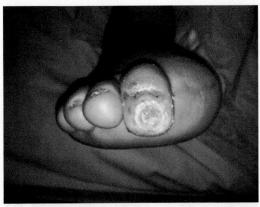

Fig. 2. Distal digital tip ulceration. Wounds commonly form on the distal aspect of digits secondary to ill-fitting shoegear or sagittal plane deformity.

extension dorsally underneath the toenail leading to onycholysis and the creation of a potential space between the nail bed and nail plate. It is the clinical experience of the authors that this represents a common but somewhat underappreciated pathway to development of infection. In our clinical practice, all distal wounds are aggressively explored to ensure that there is no extension underneath the nail plate, and the nail plate is removed in the setting of any clinical suspicion.

If an infectious process develops, then the tissue necrosis tends to initially stay locally with chronic bone necrosis of the distal phalanx, but might also eventually involve the tendinous planes of the flexor and extensor tendons. These tendons, particularly the flexor tendon, are the pathway by which infection can course proximally into the foot from the distal toes.

Distal Digital Tip: Surgical Resection and Soft Tissue Reconstruction

Complicated soft tissue reconstruction is usually not required for infectious tissue loss in this anatomic location. A portion or all of the bone of the digit is resected to a viable bone/soft tissue margin with primary closure usually easily achieved. However, it is important to investigate and decompress the remaining tendon tissue planes both dorsally and plantarly to ensure that there has been no proximal infection progression before closure. This is often done by means of the so-called "spaghetti" technique, in which the resected distal tendon ends are isolated, pulled distally, and wound around a hemostat to gain a more proximal resection margin of the tendon and decompress the remaining tendon sheath (**Fig. 3**). Depending on the specific location within the digit, different tendon patterns might be expected. Dorsally, the extensor trifurcation acts more as relatively static dorsal ligaments to the interphalangeal joints than a longitudinal and pliable tendon, because the functional insertion of the extensor tendons is into the extensor hood mechanism at the metatarsal-phalangeal joint level.[13,14] Plantarly, multiple tendons might be encountered. Surgeons should expect to see a single tendon centrally as the flexor digitorum longus that inserts onto the plantar base of the distal phalanx, but might also expect 2 tendons on either side of this, representing the split insertion of the flexor digitorum brevis onto the plantar base of the middle phalanx.

The bone might be resected at interphalangeal joint level, essentially serving as a joint disarticulation; another choice might be to remove the head and/or shaft of the

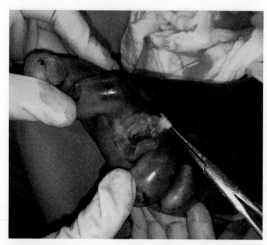

Fig. 3. Spaghetti technique for proximal tendon resection. Because tendon planes represent a common pathway for infection progression, it is important to identify, decompress, and often proximally resect tendons during excisional debridement. This is commonly done by isolating an individual tendon, pulling it distally, and winding it around a hemostat to gain a more proximal resection margin of the tendon and to relatively decompress the remaining tendon sheath.

proximal segment (leaving the phalangeal base intact) to decrease the resulting lever arm. Many find that this latter technique also has the additional benefit of being associated with more pliable soft tissue for closure. When resecting the soft tissue directly at joint level, one is likely to encounter the Grayson's and Cleland's ligaments, which attach the deep structures to the dermis.[15,16] These structures normally function to maintain the position of the skin during digital flexion and extension, but this is of course moot following amputation. However, the soft tissue between joints does not contain these structures, and is therefore more supple and pliant, and might make closure technically easier to perform.

Dorsal Interphalangeal Joint: Pathoanatomy

These ulcerations generally occur within the central digits (2, 3, and 4) and, as the result of sagittal plane digital deformity with a relatively elevated head of the proximal phalanx rubbing on shoegear (**Fig. 4**). There is very minimal soft tissue coverage between the dorsal skin and the deep tissue structures in this area, which include the extensor hood mechanism, interphalangeal joint space, head of the proximal phalanx, base of the middle phalanx, and flexor tendons in advanced cases. A similar infectious process occurs in this area as the distal digit. The tissue loss initially remains relatively local, with necrosis of the bone associated with the joint space, but may progress proximally along the course of the extensor and flexor tendons.

Interdigital, or so-called "kissing lesions," might also develop in and around the interphalangeal joints secondary to the close bone-on-bone approximation of the toes that occurs in the setting of deformity (**Fig. 5**). The pathway to infectious tissue loss here is again similar to the preceding paragraph and section.

Dorsal Interphalangeal Joint: Surgical Resection and Reconstruction

This also does not often represent a challenging soft tissue reconstruction. In a similar manner to distal digital tip ulcerations, the technically easiest procedure to perform is

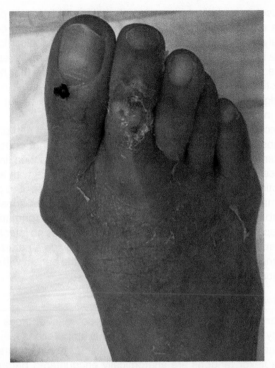

Fig. 4. Dorsal interphalangeal joint pathoanatomy. Wounds commonly form on the dorsal aspect of the proximal interphalangeal joints of the central digits secondary to sagittal plane deformity. This represents a common portal for infection and tissue loss.

a primary amputation of the digit. This might be achieved in the form of a metatarsal-phalangeal joint disarticulation, or by leaving the base of the proximal phalanx intact if viable. This latter technique might help to provide a natural spacer between adjacent digits and maintain some of the insertion of the extensor hood mechanism,

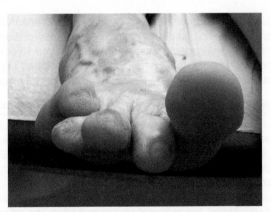

Fig. 5. Interdigital lesions pathoanatomy. Wounds commonly form between digits in the presence of deformity secondary to increased pressures caused by abnormal bone-on-bone contact.

interosseous muscles, and plantar metatarsal-phalangeal ligament/plate. This might be argued to be a more intrinsically stable anatomic construct in comparison with leaving a relatively large void following metatarsal-phalangeal disarticulation.

Once again it is important to inspect, decompress and proximally resect the remaining tendon tissue planes both dorsally and plantarly to ensure that no proximal progression of infection has occurred before closure. At this level it might also be of benefit to investigate and decompress medially and laterally about the metatarsal-phalangeal joint into the adjacent interspaces.

If the tissue necrosis is localized to the interphalangeal joint and primarily involves bone without substantial distal soft tissue loss, then one might consider performing a so-called "internal amputation" for soft tissue reconstruction in this anatomic area.[16] This is essentially similar to an arthroplasty procedure with a dorsal incision on the toe, resection of all pathologic bone and other soft tissue, and primary closure. Although the remaining toe might not be expected to maintain substantial function, this is a reasonable option if most of the soft tissue is viable (primarily evaluated by intraoperative inspection and distal capillary refill) and there is no infection progression along tendon tissue planes. At the very least this will provide a natural spacer for the adjacent tissue and avoid any negative connotations of the patient with respect to having an "amputation" performed.

Plantar Metatarsal Heads: Pathoanatomy

Increased plantar forefoot pressure from several potential sources (eg, underlying equinus deformity, plantar fat pad atrophy, previous amputations resulting in transfer lesions) might lead to a localized wound directly plantar to a metatarsal head.[17–19] In this location, the flexor tendons are anatomically encountered before the bone and represent a common course of proximal infection progression (**Fig. 6**). This occurs so frequently, in fact, that one might even argue that physicians should assume that infection is tracking toward the medial plantar vault along the flexor tendons in the setting of any acute signs or symptoms of infection, and rule it out with their examination techniques and/or advanced imaging. It is the clinical experience of the authors that the finding of epidermolysis of ulcerations in this anatomic location in a physical examination is a concern (see **Fig. 6**). Even superficial epidermolysis seems to be strongly associated with underlying infection tracking along flexor tendons toward the medial plantar vault, despite the presence of an otherwise stable appearing chronic wound.

This anatomic location is also concerning for progression of infection and tissue loss distally into the associated digit, superiorly into the metatarsal-phalangeal joint space and adjacent metatarsal-phalangeal joints, and marginally into adjacent intermetatarsal spaces. It is not uncommon, for example, for a cotton-tipped applicator to probe from a plantar metatarsal head wound straight out of the dorsal tissue.

Plantar Metatarsal Heads: Surgical Resection and Soft Tissue Reconstruction

Soft tissue reconstruction of these areas represents more of a clinical challenge because of a greater resultant soft tissue deficit, which usually follows appropriate resection. For isolated central metatarsal head tissue loss and infection, the affected soft tissue and bone might be resected either directly plantarly through the wound or through a separate dorsal incision over the metatarsal-phalangeal joint. The dorsal approach might be argued to offer the advantages of easier visualization of the resection margin of the metatarsal, the proximal phalangeal base, the adjacent metatarsal-phalangeal joints, and the adjacent interspaces. The relatively avascular plantar plate should be completely resected, and exploration, decompression, and proximal

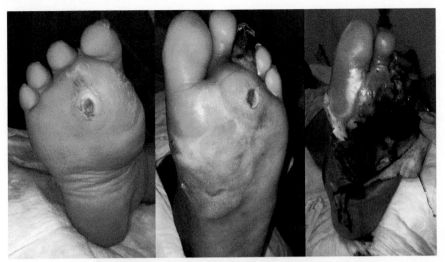

Fig. 6. Pathoanatomy of plantar metatarsal head ulcerations. Plantar metatarsal head ulcerations are a common area of pathology and infection development. It is imperative to examine for infection development along the course of the flexor digitorum longus tendons in these wounds, even in the setting of a stable appearing chronic wound (*left*). It is the experience of the authors that any epidermolysis (*center*) is a very concerning sign of infection coursing proximally along the tendon to the medial plantar vault. This tendon travels primarily within the central plantar compartment, meaning that, even in situations of severe infection (*right*), the medial and lateral plantar compartment musculature might remain viable.

resection of the extensor and flexor tendons should be performed using the "spaghetti" technique. In this anatomic location, proximal to the metatarsal-phalangeal joints, both a short and long extensor and a flexor tendon associated with each digit would be expected.[13]

Careful intraoperative attention should be directed to the course of the flexor tendons and the viability of the remaining plantar soft tissue. The flexor digitorum longus tendons travel within the central compartment of the plantar foot. This means that, even in the setting of substantial infection within the central compartment, the viability and vasculature of the medial and lateral plantar compartments might be maintained. In other words, a more proximal partial foot amputation might not be required if one is able to preserve this peripheral tissue (see **Fig. 6**). Preserved medial and lateral plantar compartments can maintain foot length and serve as a good base for soft tissue reconstruction. This is because the tissue is primarily muscular in the form of the abductor hallucis and flexor hallucis brevis muscles medially, and abductor digiti minimi muscle laterally. A local rotational flap might even be a good option for reconstruction of central compartment tissue loss.[20]

In terms of the initial plantar ulceration, one might choose to allow the wound to heal by secondary intention (as usually occurs relatively easily once the osseous prominence and pressure are removed), excise and primarily close the wound with a 3:1 ellipse, or perform a local rotational skin flap.[20–23]

Marginal plantar metatarsal head wounds (ie, the first and fifth metatarsal heads) often pose even more of a challenge for soft tissue reconstruction. Because of their eccentric location, primary closure is difficult because of the extent and specific location of the tissue loss (**Fig. 7**). Special care should be taken to assess for the viability of

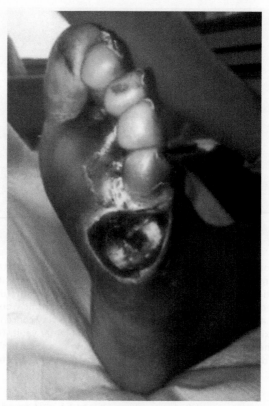

Fig. 7. Marginal plantar metatarsal head wounds. Plantar metatarsal head lesions involving the first and fifth metatarsal heads are associated with a greater degree of tissue loss and are often not easily amenable to direct primary closure.

the abductor hallucis muscle (medially) and abductor digiti minimi muscle (laterally), because this will likely determine the level of the metatarsal bone resection. In other words, in this peripheral location, there is not much advantage to leaving behind a relatively long, but viable remnant metatarsal shaft if the muscle on top of it is nonviable. For infections involving the first and fifth metatarsal heads, the authors prefer to sacrifice remnant metatarsal length for muscular coverage during closure. We have found that the length of the remaining metatarsal is less important, as long as the tendinous insertions can be maintained on the metatarsal bases. This includes the tibialis anterior tendon and peroneus longus tendon on the first metatarsal base, and the peroneus brevis tendon on the fifth metatarsal base. Although there is certainly a risk for the development of transfer lesions with partial first and fifth ray resections, we have not found this risk to be substantially increased based on a relatively long or short remnant segment. This might represent an interesting avenue for future investigation.

It is also important to appreciate that, just because the infection occurs at the level of the metatarsal-phalangeal joint, the associated digit is not necessarily a lost cause. If the soft tissue of the distal digit remains viable, then there is no need to amputate it without exemption. A similar "internal amputation" might be performed here with resection of only the metatarsal head and not the digit (**Fig. 8**). Once again the inciting ulceration might be allowed to heal by secondary intention or excised with primary closure.[16]

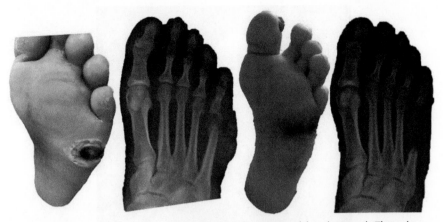

Fig. 8. Internal amputation of a marginal plantar metatarsal head wound. These images demonstrate the progression of a marginal metatarsal head wound. Initially the patient presented with an infected fifth submetatarsal head wound with clear radiographic evidence of cortical destruction. Instead of performing a partial fifth ray resection, an internal amputation of the affected bone was performed with preservation of the digit distally. The wound healed by secondary intention in a matter of weeks, maintaining the length and width of the foot.

A final option for soft tissue reconstruction of this anatomic area is by using the fillet of toe technique when the digit remains viable.[24–28] This results in amputation of the digit, but allows for use of distal viable soft tissue as a local rotational flap to help primarily close a large proximal soft tissue deficit (**Fig. 9**). This might be considered when the soft tissue deficit following a single ray amputation is so extensive that a transmetatarsal amputation is considered for closure. The procedure involves a marginal incision down the side of the digit, excision of the nail bed/plate, and removal of the phalanges of the digit, but preservation of the skin and subcutaneous tissue. This is then rotated into the soft tissue deficit and remodeled as needed depending on the specific shape of the deficit. The resulting incision often resembles a baseball, in which the dorsal foot and plantar foot are joined by rotated digital tissue.

MIDFOOT PATHOANATOMY

Primary midfoot tissue loss is relatively less common and is generally found plantarly, and associated with substantial underlying osseous deformity such as Charcot neuroarthropathy, but may also be caused by acute trauma such as a puncture wound or shoegear irritation. In this location there is relatively more soft tissue depth between the skin and deep tissue structures in comparison with the forefoot. The pathway of tissue loss and infection progression depends on the specific location of the portal, and might have a tendency to stay within a specific plantar muscular compartment (ie, medial, central, or lateral compartment) before progressing proximally or distally. In Charcot neuroarthropathy, for example, the most common location of breakdown is the plantar midfoot, with resultant osseous deformity occurring laterally under the cuboid (**Fig. 10**) or medially under one of the bones of the medial column (first metatarsal base, medial cuneiform, navicular, or talus) depending on the specific pattern of deformity (**Fig. 11**).

Laterally, physicians should appreciate that this ulceration location is in very close anatomic approximation to the peroneus longus tendon coursing around the promontory of the cuboid. In a small series of our own patients with midfoot Charcot

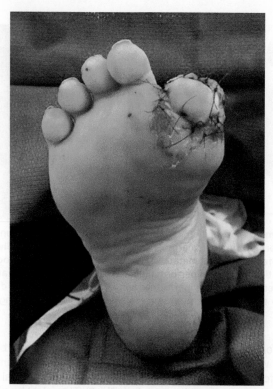

Fig. 9. Fillet of toe technique for soft tissue reconstruction of forefoot ulcerations. The fillet of toe technique involves amputation of the digit, but a local rotational flap of distal viable tissue helps close a proximal soft tissue deficit. (*Courtesy of* K. Kwaadu, DPM, Philadelphia, PA.)

neuroarthropathy (n = 14), a musculoskeletal radiologist was able to appreciate tendinopathy of the peroneus longus on magnetic resonance imaging in almost 90% of cases (see **Fig. 10**). Hence, acute infection here can quite easily traverse from the lateral to central to medial compartments of the plantar foot toward the tendon's insertion on the first metatarsal base, or proximally along the lateral rearfoot and up the lateral ankle.

Medially, the tissue loss is usually in close approximation to the abductor hallucis muscle. It is our opinion that the viability of this muscle is of the utmost importance with respect to soft tissue reconstruction. If viable, then the muscle can be used directly into any closure with local rotation, or at least indirectly as a base for tissue ingrowth. If nonviable, then a large section of tissue in the medial foot is at risk from its calcaneal origin to digital insertion. One should also be aware that communication is possible from the medial to central plantar compartments through the specific anatomy of the Knot of Henry at the crossing of the flexor hallucis longus and flexor digitorum longus tendons (see **Fig. 11**).[29]

Dorsally, substantial tissue loss might result with acute infections coursing up the extensor tendons.

MIDFOOT SURGICAL RESECTION AND SOFT TISSUE RECONSTRUCTION

Excisional debridement and surgical tissue resection in the midfoot, whether dorsally or plantarly, might result in a larger soft tissue deficit than seen in the forefoot. And to

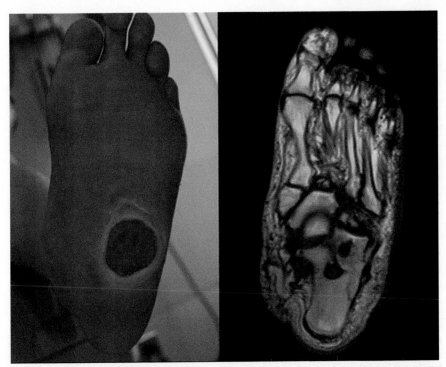

Fig. 10. Common presentation of lateral midfoot plantar tissue loss. In the setting of under-lying Charcot neuroarthropathy, chronic wounds commonly present underneath the cuboid and anterior calcaneus. Physicians should be cognizant of the close anatomic approximation of these wounds to the peroneus longus tendon, which is often affected and might serve as a portal to infection.

some degree it is less likely that direct primary closure might be achieved secondary to this. Therefore, this anatomic area is likely to be more amenable to soft tissue recon-struction involving the concepts as outlined by the reconstructive ladder. The concept of the reconstructive ladder was conceived in 1982 when Mathes and Nahai published the book *Clinical Application of Muscle and Musculocutaneous Flaps*.[30] The goal of the reconstructive ladder was to create a systematic and stepwise way of approaching complicated wound closure. Although many specific rungs on this ladder are covered in greater detail as individual articles of this edition of *Clinics*, they warrant at least a mention here.

The first rung on the ladder is basic local wound care allowing for healing by second-ary intention, essentially consisting of topical bandages and wound care products. Although saline wet-to-dry bandages were once considered a standard of wound care, contemporary advances in the form of bioengineered alternative tissues, nega-tive pressure wound therapy, and other topical treatments have essentially made this form of intervention obsolete as an initial line of therapy, except in situations of more palliative or maintenance wound care. In fact, several have instead now advocated for a concept of a reconstructive "elevator" instead of "ladder." Within this paradigm one might "skip ahead" to the most likely effective treatment as opposed to failing each individual stage before progressing to more advanced options.[31,32]

The second and third rungs on the ladder are primary wound closure and secondary (delayed) wound closure. With respect to soft tissue deficits in the setting of diabetic

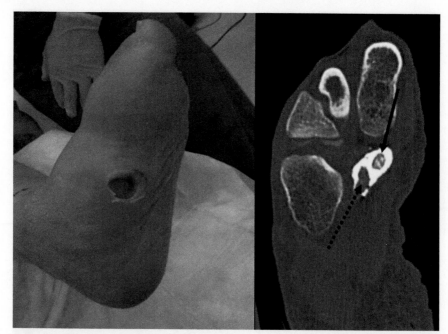

Fig. 11. Common presentation of medial midfoot plantar tissue loss. Medially physicians should be cognizant of the viability of the abductor hallucis muscle which might be used for closure, and the potential for communication of infection at the Knot of Henry between the flexor digitorum longus and flexor hallucis longus tendons.

foot disease, all infection must be resolved before closing the soft tissue envelope. For this reason, primary closure is relatively rarely performed during the first surgical intervention. Instead, the wound is packed open or left open with negative pressure wound therapy for 48 to 72 hours. If cultures remain negative and the wound does not demonstrate continued acute local signs of infection, then it might be closed during a secondary procedure. This concept of routine serial debridements approximately every 48 to 72 hours has been well studied and represents established practice at many sites.[33] Some evidence, however, has demonstrated that surgical debridement and closure as a single-stage procedure might not be detrimental as is sometimes supposed.[34]

Moving up the ladder, the next transitions are to consider split-thickness and full-thickness skin grafts. These represent a relatively efficient option for large wounds, because epithelial cells only migrate from the peripheral margin of wounds toward the center. Skin grafting allows for a relative reduction in the wound area and can dramatically decrease the physical distances that need to be covered for complete epithelialization. Although once considered too fragile for use on the weight-bearing areas of the plantar foot, more contemporary evidence has demonstrated that skin grafting might be considered even for plantar foot wounds.[35]

The final steps on the ladder are local rotational flaps, pedicled flaps, and free flaps. These are covered in greater detail in other articles of this *Clinics* edition, but it is important to consider here that these also should be considered as viable options in patients with diabetes. Patients with diabetes are certainly at increased risk for postoperative complication following foot and ankle surgery,[36] but again contemporary evidence has demonstrated that these procedures can be relatively safe and effective in this cohort.[37,38]

REARFOOT/ANKLE PATHOANATOMY

The final anatomic area of interest is the rearfoot and ankle, where potential osseous prominences include several surfaces of the calcaneus, lateral malleolus, medial malleolus, and fibular head. In these locations, the course of extrinsic tendons of the leg, which run in close approximation to these osseous structures, must be taken into consideration. Laterally, this would include the peroneus longus and peroneus brevis tendons, whereas medially this would primarily include the posterior tibial tendon and flexor digitorum longus tendon. Directly posterior, ulcerations are more likely to involve proximal extension along the Achilles and plantaris tendons.

Tissue loss in these areas is likely most commonly the result of chronic pressure in patients with a history of an acute or chronic nonambulatory state, or from an acute trauma. Particularly in nonambulatory patients, pressure ulcerations are quite common in and around the heel. Although generally this is likely to occur posteriorly, it is important to appreciate that it is probably not directly posteriorly. Most individuals have a tendency to lay with their limbs externally rotated, and therefore the tissue loss is most common on the posterior-lateral aspect of the heel, as opposed to posterior-medially or directly posteriorly.[39] This is important from an arterial inflow perspective as these locations lie in 3 different angiosomes. The more common posterior-lateral ulcerations are almost completely supplied by the peroneal artery. Assessment of this artery is often lacking, although it is certainly relatively easy to assess perfusion through this vessel by means of Doppler examination and noninvasive vascular testing.[40] Whereas posterior-medial ulcerations are within the angiosome of the posterior tibial artery, and directly posterior ulcerations are likely to have a dual flow through the posterior tibial and peroneal arteries. Just a few centimeters of anatomic space imply vastly different arterial perfusion patterns in this location.

Heel decubitus ulcerations are somewhat unlikely to occur in active, ambulating, and highly functional patients. For this reason, it is important to assess the whole patient in these clinical situations and to develop realistic mutual expectations of intervention. If a patient is nonambulatory before your intervention for a chronic heel wound, for example, it is unlikely that they will become ambulatory, even with successful reconstruction of the soft tissue. For this reason, deep tissue might be relatively aggressively resected whether from the calcaneus, distal fibula, or Achilles tendon. This level of aggressiveness with respect to deep tissue resection might help achieve direct primary closure of the soft tissue envelope.

A good example of this is with respect to partial calcanectomy procedures. Oliver and colleagues[41] recently described a technique involving resection of most of the calcaneus with direct primary closure. They reported success with this technique including having most patients able to ambulate following the procedure.

Because of the relatively large soft tissue defects that are often present, this area also represents a good opportunity for advanced techniques relatively high up the reconstructive ladder. Reverse sural flaps, for example, have been recently described for coverage of the rearfoot and ankle in the setting of diabetic tissue loss.[37,38]

SUMMARY

The primary clinical take home point for this article is for physicians to use known anatomic information to expect, and to some degree predict, the soft tissue loss that will occur with diabetic foot infections. This knowledge can be applied to minimize deficits during excisional debridement, and guide both simple and complex soft tissue closures.

One relative problem with respect to the literature on diabetic foot disease has been a lack of universally established outcome measures. In other words, is it more important that a wound heals quickly, or heals completely, or heals completely without recurrence, or heals without causing patient symptoms, or maintains patient function, or a dozen other reasonable measures? We do not claim to know the correct answer to this question, but in our practice we aim to achieve an intact soft tissue envelope as quickly as possible. Whether a wound be large or small, any wound of any size means that each morning the patient wakes up and has to deal with it in terms of dressings, bathing constraints, off-loading shoegear protocols, activity limitations, driving restrictions, frequent physician visits, long courses of antibiotics, and so forth. Only once the soft tissue envelope is intact can the patient begin a return to relative normalcy.

REFERENCES

1. van Netten JJ, Price PE, Lavery LA, et al. Prevention of foot ulcers in the at-risk patient with diabetes. Diabetes Metab Res Rev 2016;32(Suppl 1):84–98.
2. Dorreteijn JA, Kriegsman DM, Assendelft WJ, et al. Patient education for preventing diabetic foot ulceration. Cochrane Database Syst Rev 2010;12(5):CD001488.
3. Singh N, Armstrong DG, Lipsky BA. Preventing foot ulcers in patients with diabetes. JAMA 2005;293(2):217–28.
4. Schaper NC, Van Netten JJ, Apelqvist J, et al. Prevention and management of foot problems in diabetes: a summary guidance for daily practice 2015, based on the IWGDF guidance documents. Diabetes Metab Res Rev 2016;32(Suppl 1):7–15.
5. Driver VR, Fabbi M, Lavery L, et al. The costs of diabetic foot: the economic case for the limb salvage team. J Vasc Surg 2010;52(Suppl):17S–22S.
6. Hunt NA, Liu GT, Lavery LA. The economics of limb salvage in diabetes. Plast Reconstr Surg 2011;127(Suppl 1):289S–95S.
7. Bibbo C, Ehrlich D, Levin LS, et al. Maintaining levels of lower extremity amputations. J Surg Orthop Adv 2016;25(3):137–48.
8. Markakis K, Bowling FL, Boulton AJ. The diabetic foot in 2015: an overview. Diabetes Metab Res Rev 2016;32(Suppl 1):169–78.
9. Pickwell K, Siersma VD, Holstein PE, et al. Diabetic foot disease: impact of ulcer location on ulcer healing. Diabetes Metab Res Rev 2013;29(5):377–83.
10. Ledoux WR, Shofer JB, Cowley MS, et al. Diabetic foot ulcer incidence in relation to plantar pressure magnitude and measurement location. J Diabetes Complications 2013;27(6):621–6.
11. Faglia E, Clerici G, Caminiti M, et al. Influence of osteomyelitis location in the foot of diabetic patients with transtibial amputation. Foot Ankle Int 2013;34(2):222–7.
12. Borkosky SL, Roukis TS. Incidence of repeat amputation after partial first ray amputation associated with diabetes mellitus and peripheral neuropathy: an 11-year review. J Foot Ankle Surg 2013;52(3):335–8.
13. Sarrafian SK. Tendon sheaths and bursae. In: Sarrafian SK, editor. Anatomy of the foot and ankle: Descriptive, topographical, functional. Philadelphia: J.B. Lippincott Company; 1983. p. 251–60.
14. Zwanenburg RL, McGrouther DA, Werker PMN. Grayson ligament: a revised description of its anatomy and function. J Hand Surg Am 2018. https://doi.org/10.1016/j.jhsa.2018.07.002.

15. Zwanenburg RL, Werker PM, McGrouther DA. The anatomy and function of Cleland's ligaments. J Hand Surg Eur Vol 2014;39(5):482–90.
16. Falgia E, Clerici G, Caminiti M, et al. Feasibility and effectiveness of internal pedal amputation of phalanx or metatarsal head in diabetic patients with forefoot osteomyelitis. J Foot Ankle Surg 2012;51(5):593–8.
17. Aragon-Sanchez J, Lazaro-Martinez JL, Pulido-Duque J, et al. From the diabetic foot ulcer and beyond: how do foot infections spread in patients with diabetes? Diabet Foot Ankle 2012;3:18693.
18. Dalal S, Widgerow A, Evans GRD. The plantar fat pad and the diabetic foot – a review. Int Wound J 2015;12(6):636–40.
19. Cunha M, Faul J, Steinberg J, et al. Forefoot ulcer recurrence following partial first ray amputation: the role of tendo-Achilles lengthening. J Am Podiatr Med Assoc 2010;100(1):80–2.
20. Boffeli TJ, Reinking R. Plantar rotational flap technique for panmetatarsal head resection and transmetatarsal amputation: a revision approach for second metatarsal head transfer ulcers in patients with previous partial first ray amputation. J Foot Ankle Surg 2014;53(1):96–100.
21. Boffeli TJ, Hyllengren SB. Unilobed rotational flap for plantar hallux interphalangeal joint ulceration complicated by osteomyelitis. J Foot Ankle Surg 2015; 54(6):1166–71.
22. Ramanujam CL, Zgonis T. Use of local flaps for soft-tissue closure in diabetic foot wounds: a systematic review. Foot Ankle Spec 2018;. https://doi.org/10.1177/1938640018803745.
23. Rosenblum BI, Giurini JM, Miller LB, et al. Neuropathic ulcerations plantar to the lateral column in patients with Charcot foot deformity: a flexible approach to lib salvage. J Foot Ankle Surg 1997;36(5):360–3.
24. Kuntscher MV, Erdmann D, Homann HH, et al. The concept of fillet flaps: classification, indications, and analysis of their clinical value. Plast Reconstr Surg 2001; 108(4):885–96.
25. Schade VL. Digital fillet flaps: a systematic review. Foot Ankle Spec 2015;8(4): 273–8.
26. Chung SR, Wong KL, Cheah AE. The lateral lesser toe fillet flap for diabetic foot soft tissue closure: surgical technique and case report. Diabet Foot Ankle 2014;5: 25732.
27. Baek SO, Suh HW, Lee JY. Modified toe pulp fillet flap coverage: better wound healing and satisfactory length preservation. Arch Plast Surg 2018;45(1):62–8.
28. Aerden D, Vanmierlo B, Denecker N, et al. Primary closure with a filleted hallux flap after transmetatarsal amputation of the big toe for osteomyelitis in the diabetic foot: a short series of four cases. Int J Low Extrem Wounds 2012;11(2):80–4.
29. Ali S, Griffin NL, Ellis W, et al. Communication of contrast in the flexor hallucis longus tendon with other pedal tendons at the Master Knot of Henry. J Am Podiatr Med Assoc 2017;107(2):166–70.
30. Mathes S, Nahai F. Clinical application for muscle and musculocutaneous flaps. St Louis (MO): Mosby; 1982. p. 3.
31. Glat P, Davenport T. Current techniques for burn reconstruction: using dehydrated human amnion/chorion membrane allografts as an adjunctive treatment along the reconstructive ladder. Ann Plast Surg 2017;78(Suppl 1):S14–8.
32. Janis JE, Kwon RK, Attinger CE. The new reconstructive ladder: modifications to the traditional model. Plast Reconstr Surg 2011;127(Suppl 1):205S–12S.

33. Cardinal M, Eisenbud DE, Armstrong DG, et al. Serial surgical debridement: a retrospective study on clinical outcomes in chronic lower extremity wounds. Wound Repair Regen 2009;17(3):306–11.
34. Blume PA, Paragas LK, Sumpio BE, et al. Single-stage surgical treatment of noninfected diabetic foot ulcers. Plast Reconstr Surg 2002;109(2):601–9.
35. Rose JF, Giovinco N, Mills JL, et al. Split-thickness skin grafting the high-risk diabetic foot. J Vasc Surg 2014;59(6):1657–63.
36. Wukich DK, Lowery NJ, McMillen RL, et al. Postoperative infection rates in foot and ankle surgery: a comparison of patients with and without diabetes mellitus. J Bone Joint Surg Am 2010;92(2):287–95.
37. Morgan K, Brantigan CO, Field CJ, et al. Reverse sural artery flap for the reconstruction of chronic lower extremity wounds in high-risk patients. J Foot Ankle Surg 2006;45(6):417–23.
38. Ignatiadis IA, Tsiampa VA, Galanakos SP, et al. The reverse sural fasciocutaneous flap for the treatment of traumatic, infectious or diabetic foot and ankle wounds: a retrospective review of 16 patients. Diabet Foot Ankle 2011;2. https://doi.org/10.3402/dfa.v2i0.5653.
39. Crowell A, Meyr AJ. Accuracy of the ankle-brachial index in the assessment of arterial perfusion of heel pressure injuries. Wounds 2017;29(2):51–5.
40. Ellis-McConnell W, Taylor A, Kelly P, et al. Quantitative assessment of peroneal artery pressure at the ankle with noninvasive vascular testing. J Foot Ankle Surg 2017;56(3):551–4.
41. Oliver NG, Steinberg JS, Powers K, et al. Lower extremity function following partial calcanectomy in high-risk limb salvage patients. J Diabetes Res 2015;2015:432164.

Pedicled and Free Tissue Transfers

Cara K. Black, BA[a], Vikas S. Kotha, BS[a], Kenneth L. Fan, MD[a],
Kevin Ragothaman, DPM[b], Christopher E. Attinger, MD[a], Karen Kim Evans, MD[a],*

KEYWORDS

- Flap • Local muscle flap • Free flap • Complex foot wound
- Flexor digitorum brevis flap • Abductor digiti minimi flap • Abductor hallucis flap
- Tissue defect

KEY POINTS

- Complex wounds that are the sequalae of diabetic foot disease often require complex soft-tissue rearrangement to achieve closure and maintain a functional limb.
- Local and intrinsic muscle flaps are viable options for small defects with exposed bone or tendon that are within reach of the muscle of interest.
- Free flaps are beneficial for large tissue defects and have been proven to provide superb durability.
- Postoperative flap monitoring is essential to ensure flap viability and appropriate management of complications.

INTRODUCTION

The lifetime risk of developing a foot ulcer is approximately 15% to 20% for patients with diabetes, and has surpassed diabetic coma as the primary driver of mortality in diabetes.[1-3] The burden on the health care system is significant: approximately 25% to 33% of the total cost of diabetes on the health care system is spent on lower extremity ulcers.[4] Rates have steadily increased, and hospitalizations for amputations doubled from 33,000 in 1980 to 71,000 in 2005. Five-year mortality rates for new-onset diabetic ulcers are between 43% and 55% and increase to 75% after amputation.[5] The causative progression of diabetic foot wounds to amputation is extensively documented and is preceded by a combination of ischemia, infection, neuropathy,

Disclosure Statement: The authors have nothing to disclose.
[a] Department of Plastic and Reconstructive Surgery, MedStar Georgetown University Hospital, 3800 Reservoir Road, Washington, DC 20007, USA; [b] Division of Podiatric Surgery, MedStar Georgetown University, 3800 Reservoir Road, Washington, DC 20007, USA
* Corresponding author. Department of Plastic and Reconstructive Surgery, Center for Wound Healing and Hyperbaric Medicine, MedStar Georgetown University Hospital, 3800 Reservoir Road, One Bles, Washington, DC 20007.
E-mail address: karen.k.evans@gunet.georgetown.edu

Clin Podiatr Med Surg 36 (2019) 441–455
https://doi.org/10.1016/j.cpm.2019.03.002
0891-8422/19/© 2019 Elsevier Inc. All rights reserved.

podiatric.theclinics.com

and initial minor trauma.[6] In more than 86% of limbs, a preventable sentinel event preceded amputation. Prevention of amputation is possible and critical with a multidisciplinary team, by using aggressive wound coverage and revascularization modalities to existing wounds and prevention of future wounds.[4] In this setting, amputations may be reduced up to 82%, leading to both cost and mortality benefit.[7–9] Furthermore, lower extremity microvascular free tissue transfer (FTT) is significantly associated with a higher 5-year survival rate in comparison with patients who undergo amputations.[10–12]

As such, local or free flaps are instrumental in salvage of complex wounds in the diabetic foot. Traditionally the reconstructive ladder is used to conceptualize the incremental thought process behind reconstructive solutions. However, the lower rungs of the ladder, such as primary closure or skin grafting, are often inadequate in the lower extremity because of the lack of available local soft-tissue, the stress of ambulation, and the inadequate recipient bed. In addition, the focus on achieving optimal functional outcomes, improving donor site appearance, and reducing morbidity has led to a focus on local and FTT to meet reconstructive needs.[13] Flaps are transferred units of tissue that have their own blood supply; whereas grafts rely on vessel ingrowth at the recipient bed. Flaps in the setting of foot reconstruction are usually composed of skin, subcutaneous tissue, and muscle, but may occasionally have an osseous segment. Local or pedicled flaps lie within the proximity of the wound, either adjacent or interpolated, and are designed to preserve the tissue's blood supply. FTT occurs when a unit of tissue with its corresponding vessels are disinserted from a source vessel and subsequently reanastomosed to a recipient artery and vein in a distant wound bed using a microsurgical technique. In other words, it is the autotransplantation of isolated tissue from one area of the body to a distant site.

Flap coverage is the reconstructive choice for ulcers and defects with exposed tendons, joints, or bone. Flaps should only be used after thorough debridement of all nonviable soft-tissue and bone to remove infectious agents, biofilm, and/or senescent cells that impede normal wound healing.[14] Generally speaking, the size of the defect determines whether or not a local flap can be used.[12] In the case of smaller defects (approximately 3 × 6 cm or less), a local flap is usually used when available. Larger defects or those out of reach of local flaps usually require a free flap. However, some researchers advocate proceeding directly to FTT in limb salvage to restore optimum form and function if there are prerequisite surgeon and institutional capabilities.[13,15,16] In the authors' series, 86.1% of diabetic wounds salvaged with FTT were ambulating at 1.53 years (Black et al, unpublished data, 2019).

Consideration of blood supply is of utmost importance when planning any reconstruction. A renaissance in reconstructive surgery occurred with the work of Macgregor and Morgan[17] on the anatomic basis of local skin flaps in 1973. They categorized local cutaneous flaps based on their blood supply, proposing 4 major types of local skin flaps: random flaps without a source vessel based on the subdermal plexus; axial flaps based on a single source artery within the longitudinal axis of the flap; reverse axial flaps whereby the source vessel is divided proximally and blood flows in a retrograde fashion; and island flaps whereby flaps are based solely on the pedicle devoid of intervening skin segments. In 1987 Taylor and Palmer[18] identified 40 separate units of skin on the human body, known as angiosomes, supplied by a single source artery, linked by to each other by either true anastomotic arteries or choke vessels. Occluding a source artery dilates choke vessels, which serves as the surgical basis of the "delay phenomenon," whereby surgeons ligate vessels in preparation for future transfer.[19] Nakajima and colleagues,[20] in the most comprehensive classification system, organized the origins of these source vessels into 6 categories and 2 overall subtypes, direct and indirect perforating vessels (**Table 1**).

Table 1 Nakajima subtypes of fasciocutaneous flaps	
Type I (A)	Direct cutaneous vessels
Type II (B)	Direct septocutaneous vessels
Type III (C)	Direct cutaneous branch of muscular vessels
Type IV (D)	Perforating cutaneous branch of muscular vessels (indirect)
Type V (E)	Septocutaneous perforator (direct)
Type VI (F)	Musculocutaneous perforator (indirect)

Considered a classic, this underappreciated classification system has withstood the test of time, aiding the reconstructive surgeon in conceptualizing the entire spectrum of varied anatomy of vascular pedicles (**Fig. 1**).[21] When considering muscle flaps, Mathes and Nahai[22] determined that muscles have differing prerequisite blood supply (**Table 2**). Some muscles are able to survive entirely off a single dominant vessel (types I, II, III, and V), whereas other muscles can survive off of vessels segmentally perfusing each portion of the muscle (types IV and V). Consideration of the blood supply allows surgeons to delineate which vessels may be sacrificed from those vessels that are imperative for reconstructive success so that a muscle flap can be transferred into the wound without compromise.

To further our understanding of the vascular anatomy of the foot, the senior authors (C.E.A. and K.K.E.) identified 6 angiosomes of the foot and ankle, all originating from the 3 main arteries of the lower leg.[23] Application of the angiosome theory is important in reconstructive success of the foot. Incisions should be placed between angiosomes to limit perfusion compromise (eg, slightly above glabrous junctions medially, at the glabrous junction laterally, and midline sagittally on the plantar and posterior aspect). Knowledge will help guide the surgeon in determining which amputations and skin flaps will heal. A vascular surgeon can use this knowledge to bring blood supply to

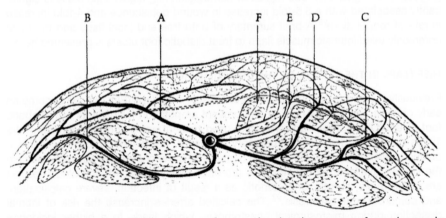

Fig. 1. Nakajima pattern of deep fascia perforators showing the concept of vascular supply to the skin, and classification of flaps based on their vascularization type. These are the 6 patterns of the vascular supply to the fasciocutaneous plexus. Type A: direct cutaneous vessel; type B: direct septocutaneous vessel; type C: direct cutaneous branch of muscular vessel; type D: perforating cutaneous branch of muscular vessel; type E: septocutaneous perforator; type F: musculocutaneous perforator. (*Reproduced from* Nakajima H, Fujino T, Adachi S. A new concept of vascular supply to the skin and classification of skin flaps according to their vascularization. Ann Plast Surg 1986;16(1):1–19 (Figure 2); with permission.)

Table 2	
Mathes and Nahai classification of muscle flap blood supply	
Type I	Single vascular pedicle
Type II	Dominant pedicle(s) and minor pedicle(s) (i.e., abductor digiti minimi flap, abductor hallucis muscle flap)
Type III	Two dominant pedicles
Type IV	Segmental vascular pedicles
Type V	Single dominant pedicle and secondary segmental pedicles

ischemic ulcers during revascularization. Furthermore, the application of the angio-some theory can dictate which pedicled local options are available.

Three distinct angiosomes of the plantar foot are supplied by 3 branches of the posterior tibial (PT) artery: the calcaneal branch of the PT artery feeds the medial and plantar heel, the medial plantar artery (MPA) feeds the plantar instep, and the lateral plantar artery (LPA) feeds the lateral midfoot and forefoot. Two angiosomes are located on the anterolateral portion of the ankle and rear foot and are supplied by the 2 branches of the peroneal artery: the calcaneal branch of the peroneal artery feeds the lateral and plantar heel, and the anterior perforating branch of the peroneal artery feeds the anterolateral ankle. Finally, the anterior tibial artery (and its continuation after crossing the ankle, the dorsalis pedis artery) supplies the final angiosome over the anterior ankle and dorsum of the foot.

The authors' diabetic foot ulcer management algorithm (**Fig. 2**) before reconstruction relies on a multidisciplinary approach with surgical debridement to achieve a culture-negative wound bed, angiography to define available vasculature and facilitate endovascular therapies, vein studies to identify the availability of superficial and deep veins, and hypercoagulable studies to determine propensity for perioperative flap thrombosis.[24] Critical to this discussion is preoperative and perioperative glucose control: glucose level higher than 200 mg/dL or hemoglobin A_{1C} higher than 6.5% is significantly associated with a 3.5-fold increase in wound dehiscence and 4-fold increase in rate of reoperation.[25] A brief summary of both free and local flaps and the most commonly used intrinsic muscle flaps to treat diabetic foot ulcers is presented here.

FREE FLAPS IN THE SETTING OF THE DIABETIC LIMB

Previously thought of as a treatment of last resort, free flaps (**Fig. 3**) have become an early option to accelerate healing and prevent amputation for patients with diabetic foot ulcers (DFUs). Free flaps were first used to treat ankle and foot defects in the 1970s during the dawn of microsurgery. However, the diabetic patient presents a unique challenge for free flaps with a higher rate of reconstructive failure[26] because the vessels available for anastomosis are often highly diseased. The blood vessels are often fragile, fibrotic, and stenotic as a result of infection, severe calcification, and comorbid atherosclerosis.[27] The calcified arteries increase the risk of intimal dissection during microsurgical anastomosis, which leads to a higher incidence of thrombosis and complications.[28] Patients also often have limited blood supply to the lower extremity, hindering the number of recipient vessels available for anastomosis.

When considering anastomotic technique of the flap to the recipient vessels, the limited blood supply precludes end-to-end anastomosis, whereby a major artery of the leg is cut and rerouted to the flap. The ischemic extremity requires an end-to-side microsurgical technique to preserve native vasculature. In the setting of severely

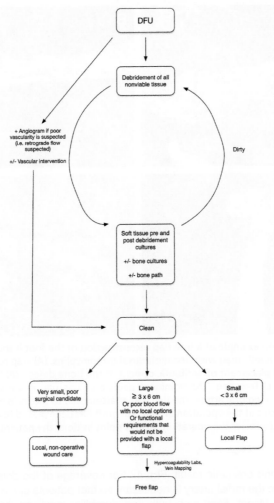

Fig. 2. Algorithmic reconstructive approach to the patient with a diabetic foot ulcer (DFU).

calcific arteries, the senior author (K.K.E.) uses a novel end-to-side interpositional saphenous vein patch to eliminate outside to in suturing in calcific vessels, decreasing the risk of intimal fracture.[29] With careful consideration of technique, diabetic patients can experience flap survival rates of 93%, limb salvage rates between 79% and 90%, and amputation-free 1-year survival rates of approximately 82%.[30,31] The most common flap used flap at the authors' institution is the ipsilateral anterolateral thigh (ALT) or the vastus lateralis (VL) flap based off of the descending branch of the lateral femoral circumflex artery, owing to the low morbidity of removing a part of the muscle without sacrificing upper extremity or core strength.[32] The alternatives, such as the free rectus flap or the latissimus dorsi flap, need to be preserved to maintain upper body strength should an amputation be necessary. When selecting a flap, the needs of the area to be reconstructed should be considered. A useful approach is the subunit principle of the foot described by Hollenbeck and colleagues.[16] The authors defined 7 subunits and recommended free flaps that would provide the

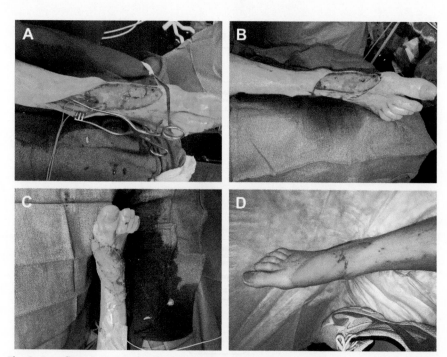

Fig. 3. Free flap. An example of a free flap reconstruction of the foot is shown. The patient is a 57-year-old diabetic man with first metatarsal osteomyelitis. (*A*) Flap recipient site after debridement and placement of antibiotic cement in the bone defect. (*B*) Placement of the vastus lateralis (VL) free flap. The dominant pedicle of this flap is the lateral circumflex branch of the deep femoral artery. The flap was anastomosed to the recipient anterior tibial vessels. (*C*) End result of the operation after a skin graft has been placed to cover the VL free flap. (*D*) Eight weeks after the operation. At this point in time, the patient was ambulating in a regular shoe.

best functional and cosmetic result (**Fig. 4**). For coverage of the dorsum, a thin flap such as one from the radial artery is necessary so that patients can eventually fit into shoes. For heel ulcers, flaps with bulk and durability, such as the ALT or VL, is required. The authors showed an excellent limb salvage rate of 89% and free flap survival rate of 92% when using this approach to planning. Because of the documented success, free flaps are an excellent option for larger foot defects to promote wound coverage. Furthermore, flaps provide new blood supply to improve healing and vasculogenesis in the ischemic DFU.

LOCAL FLAPS IN THE SETTING OF THE DIABETIC LIMB
Introduction to Local Flaps

Local flaps were first pioneered by Ger[33–36] in the late 1960s. Their development was based on the principle that the rotation of well-vascularized muscle to cover soft-tissue defects improved local blood flow and provided a hospitable surface for a skin graft. The intrinsic muscles of the foot are all classified as Mathes and Nahai type II flap muscles because they have one dominant proximal vascular pedicle and one or more distal minor pedicles.[37] This is relevant to our understanding of local flap success because even though the major pedicle is maintained in flap rotation, the flap muscle can also survive on more distal minor pedicles.[37–39]

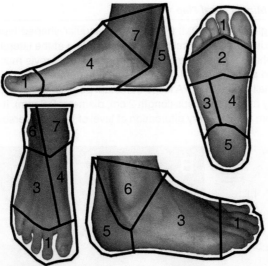

Subunit	Demands: Tissue Needs	Optimal Flaps
1	Low functional, Moderate aesthetic: small, thin and pliable.	Radial forearm > lateral arm
2	High functional, Low aesthetic: durable and minimal bulk.	([a]): Radial forearm > lateral arm > gracilis with STSG > ALT
3 / 4	Low functional, High aesthetic: smooth, thin and pliable.	Radial forearm > ALT > scapular > latissimus dorsi
5	High functional, Low aesthetic: durable and moderate bulk.	([a]): ALT > gracilis with STSG > latissimus dorsi > scapular >lateral arm > radial forearm
6 / 7	Moderate functional, Moderate aesthetic: may vary from smooth, thin and pliable to large and bulky.	Gracilis with STSG, latissimus dorsi, ALT, rectus abdominis, lateral arm, radial forearm, scapular

Fig. 4. Subunit approach to foot reconstruction. Four views of the foot and ankle are shown with 7 functionally and aesthetically different subunits. The table indicates the unique tissue demands and optimal flaps for each subunit. STSG, split-thickness skin graft; ALT, anterolateral thigh. [a] Nerve coaptation may be considered. (*From* Hollenbeck ST, Woo S, Komatsu I, et al. Longitudinal outcomes and application of the subunit principle to 165 foot and ankle free tissue transfers. Plast Reconstr Surg 2010;125(3):924–34; with permission.)

Local pedicled flaps provide a simpler and successful alternative to FTT for small (<3 × 6 cm) defects of the foot and ankle with exposed bone (with or without osteomyelitis), joint, or tendon.[37] The senior author (C.E.A.) previously found that diabetes does not affect the viability of local pedicled flaps, with limb salvage and healing rates similar to those of trauma patients.[12,37] However, diabetic patients had a 2-fold increase in healing time, 2.7-fold increase in hospital length of stay, and lower long-term survival (63% in diabetic patients versus 100% in the trauma group). In this cohort, limb salvage prolonged survival of diabetic patients.[12,37] In a retrospective noninferiority trial, the senior author demonstrated local flaps were equivalent to FTT in treatment of local soft-tissue defects, with no difference in complication rates or flap success.[12,37] Although local flaps require a shorter operating time and lower immediate costs than free flaps, some investigators have found that use of pedicled flaps results in a higher overall complication rate (36%–45% for local flaps versus 16%–30% for free flaps).[40,41] Overall the differences may be surgeon dependent, and local flaps should be considered a viable option in diabetic foot reconstruction.

Abductor Digiti Minimi Local Flap

The abductor digiti minimi (ADM) (**Fig. 5**) is a triangular-shaped type II muscle originating at the medial and lateral calcaneus and inserting at the lateral side of the small toe's proximal phalanx alongside the flexor digiti minimi brevis muscles. The bulk of the ADM is found at the proximal portion of the fifth metatarsal, as the muscle serves to abduct the small toe.[42] The LPA is the dominant pedicle, which enters the muscle at its origin medially at the calcaneus (length 2 cm, diameter 0.6 mm). It originates alongside the MPA from the PT artery bifurcation at level of the transverse septum between

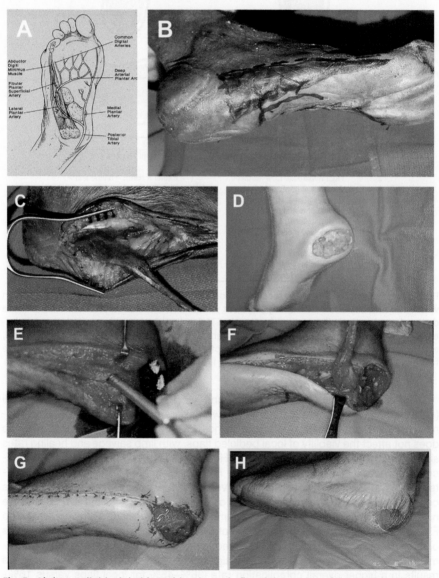

Fig. 5. Abductor digiti minimi (ADM) local muscle flap. (*A*) Drawing of the ADM local muscle flap. (*B*) Flap markings. (*C*) Flap isolated on its dominant pedicle, the lateral plantar artery. Note the small distal bulk. (*D–H*) ADM flap coverage of calcaneal osteomyelitis.

the abductor hallucis longus and flexor digitorum brevis muscles. Preoperatively, a palpable PT pulse should be obtained to reassure plantar lateral perfusion.

The ADM muscle flap, on average 10 cm long and 3 cm wide, is useful for calcaneal osteomyelitis, plantar heel defects, lateral ankle defects, and even midfoot reconstruction.[43] The ADM is released from its distal insertion into the fifth digit proximal phalanx and dissection is carried proximally, taking care to gently separate the ADM from the flexor hallucis brevis muscle belly. The flap has 1 to 2 minor pedicles that are ligated. The major vascular pedicle lies proximal to the fifth metatarsal styloid process and should be preserved. Although rare, elevating a musculocutaneous pedicled flap is possible.[42] The ADM muscle flap is relatively small and has a small arc of rotation. Disorigination at the lateral calcaneus may increase mobilization if needed. For larger defects, the ADM flap can be combined with the abductor hallucis (AH) flap for heel coverage or extensor digitorum brevis flap for lateral malleolus coverage.[43]

Following flap inset, skin grafting the flap can be helpful. Primary closure is sufficient for the donor site, and negative pressure therapy for the first week after surgery can help improve skin graft take and healing. It is imperative that the ankle is immobilized so the suture line is not affected. The flap should be protected with a splint, boot, or cast. Patients should remain non–weight bearing for a month after surgery and be counseled that poor blood glucose control and vasoconstrictive substances can lead to flap loss. As long as this care is taken, this flap is highly survivable.

Abductor Hallucis Local Flap

A type II muscle with 2 to 3 minor pedicles, the AH originates from the calcaneus and inserts into the medial aspect of the hallux's proximal phalanx (**Fig. 6**). It serves to support the medial longitudinal arch and enables abduction and flexion of the hallux. The muscle is supplied by an approximately 2-cm-long, 0.6-mm-diameter major pedicle derived from the proximal, deep branch of the MPA, a continuation of the PT artery. The major pedicle runs along the medial intramuscular septum between the AH and flexor brevis muscles. It can be extended up to 3 cm if needed. Venous drainage and motor and sensory innervation are provided by lateral plantar comitantes and the medial plantar nerve, respectively. Preoperatively, a palpable PT pulse should be obtained to reassure medial plantar perfusion.[42]

AH muscle flaps (10 cm long × 3 cm wide) can be reliably harvested and superiorly rotated to cover wounds of the medial heel, ankle, and, if needed, the midfoot. For large midfoot and plantar heel defects, combining AH and ADM flaps can be helpful. The pivot point is the distal tarsal tunnel. Because the major pedicle is located proximally at the distal tarsal tunnel, it is safe to ligate distal pedicles for viable distal-to-proximal rotation of the flap. If needed, distal foot coverage is possible but less reliable; disoriginating the AH at the medial calcaneus can increase the arc of rotation to cover the metatarsals, for example.[42] It should be noted that the distal insertion of AH is tendinous and may be unsuitable for distal wound coverage. To increase flap bulk, the muscle can be raised with an MPA fasciocutaneous flap in order to perform a distal arc rotation.

To prevent hallux valgus, tenodesis of the AH tendon to the medial metatarsal should be done. Following flap inset, skin graft loss can be minimized by avoiding tendon grafting. Primary donor site closure and postoperative care similar to that of the ADM flap are adequate.

Flexor Digitorum Brevis Local Flap

The flexor digitorum brevis (FDB) muscle flap (**Fig. 7**) is another useful local flap in the diabetic patient. The FDB muscle lies deep to the plantar fascia between the AH and

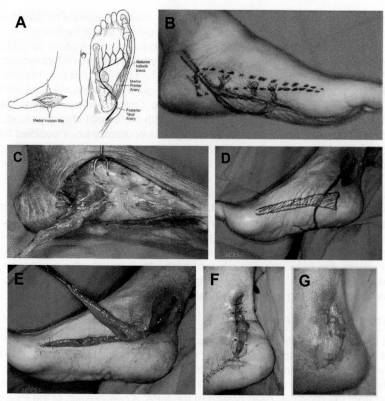

Fig. 6. Abductor hallucis (AH) local muscle flap. (*A*) Drawing of the AH local muscle flap. (*B*) Flap markings. (*C*) Flap isolated on its dominant pedicle, the medial plantar artery. (*D–G*) AH flap coverage of a nonhealing ulcer over the Achilles tendon. ([A] *From* Attinger CE, Clemens MW. Foot and ankle reconstruction. In: Thorne CH, editor. Grabb and Smith's plastic surgery, 7th edition. Philadelphia: Wolters Kluwer; 2014; with permission.)

ADM and enables toe flexion. It originates from the medial calcaneal process and plantar fascia and inserts onto the 2nd-5th toe middle phalanges. Dominant blood supply is provided by the proximal branches of the LPA, which after entering the middle foot compartment travels obliquely toward the 5th metatarsal between the FDB and quadratus plantar muscle. The LPA, as well as branches of the MPA, supply 2 to 3 minor pedicles each. Both dominant pedicles are on average 1 to 2 cm long and 0.6 mm in diameter. As with AH and ADM flaps, a palpable preoperative PT pulse should be obtained to reassure perfusion.[42] The venae comitantes of the LPA and MPA drain venous blood to the PT veins. Sensory innervation is provided by branches of the calcaneal nerve, lateral plantar nerve, and medial plantar nerve, which also provides motor innervation.

Like the AH, the FDB is primarily used as a motor muscle flap with an average length of 10 cm and width of 4 cm. This flap is a good option for small wounds of the plantar heel because it has a 180° arc of rotation around its pivot point, the distal plantar heel.[42] However, sufficient pedicle dissection can allow the flap to reach the Achilles tendon. Because it is small, its best utility is with deep defects that can be covered primarily with local glabrous skin. During elevation, it is helpful to suture the 4 flexor tendons together after they are divided distally. If distal wound coverage is needed, a

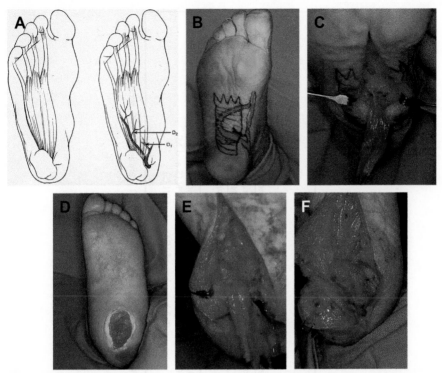

Fig. 7. Flexor digitorum brevis (FDB) muscle local flap. (*A*) Drawing of the FDB muscle local flap. D1, branch of the medial plantar artery (MPA); D2, lateral plantar artery (LPA). (*B*) Flap markings. (*C*) Flap isolated on its dominant pedicle, the LPA. (*D–F*) Flap coverage of a non-healing ulcer on the plantar aspect of the foot secondary to overlengthening of the Achilles tendon.

reverse flap can be designed as long as distal plantar arch perfusion is sufficient. FDB flaps can be muscle only, or musculocutaneous (V-Y advancement flap allowing 2–3 cm of advancement) with a skin area of 12 cm length by 5 cm width. If a skin island is taken, it should lie adjacent to the non–weight-bearing 2nd-4th metatarsals.

The plantar fascia should be carefully reapproximated before closure. Primary closure with a small drain removed the day after surgery is sufficient for the donor site. Postoperative elevation is important to avoid fluid accumulation. Patients may ambulate with crutches with strict non–weight-bearing status regarding the operated limb, but if noncompliant the foot may be immobilized with an external fixator frame for 3 to 4 weeks after surgery until ambulation is safe.

Dressing and Postoperative Flap Care

It is critical to attain intraoperative hemostasis to reduce the risk of postoperative complications, including development of hematoma or edema, and insertion of a drain may be required. Following minimal tension closure with nonabsorbable suture and staples, a nonadherent dressing is applied to the flap. A bulky padded dressing is applied to minimize pressure and shear on the flap. Incisional negative pressure therapy dressing can be applied to the wound to minimize tension of the closure in the postoperative period when edema can occur.[44] An external fixator can be applied for the

Table 3
Summary of most common local foot flaps

Local Flap	Arterial Supply	Venous Supply	Major Pedicle (Length/Diameter)	Minor Pedicle (Length/Diameter)	Innervation	Primarily Used For
Abductor digiti minimi	LPA	LPA venae comitantes	LPA (2 cm/0.6 mm)	LPA (1 cm/0.5 mm)	Sural nerve (S) LPN (S and M)	Small lateral foot defects
Abductor hallucis	Proximal branch of MPA	LPA venae comitantes	MPA (2 cm/0.6 mm)	2–3 branches of MPA (1.5 cm/0.5 mm)	MPN (S and M)	Small medial foot defects
Flexor digitorum brevis	Proximal branches of MPA and LPA	LPA venae comitantes	MPA (1–2 cm/0.6 mm) LPA (1–2 cm/0.6 mm)	2–3 branches of MPA (1 cm/0.5 mm) 2–3 branches of LPA (1 cm/0.5 mm)	Calcaneal nerve (S) MPN (S and M) LPN (S)	Small heel defects

Abbreviations: LPA, lateral plantar artery; LPN, lateral plantar nerve; M, motor; MPA, medial plantar artery; MPN, medial plantar nerve; S, sensory purpose of postoperative offloading. It is imperative that patients are non–weight bearing to the operative limb.

All flaps should be monitored carefully after surgery. The flap should be routinely examined for color or temperature change and signs of infection. A pale color or coldness to the touch with the dorsum of the examiner's hand indicates a possible lack of arterial flow to the flap and should be verified with Doppler examination. Darkening of the flap could indicate venous congestion. In the setting of free flaps, prompt operative management with interrogation of the anastomosis is critical. In the setting of local flaps, the authors generally will place the flap back into the original defect to take advantage of the delay phenomenon. In 7 to 10 days, when the flap vessel and the choke vessels have dilated, the flap is placed into the wound. Arterial perfusion may be verified by indocyanine green angiography. Adjuncts such as nitroglycerin paste and hyperbaric oxygen may be used in the setting of compromised vascularity, but are rarely the primary modality.

SUMMARY

Preserving the integrity of the diabetic foot is crucial because in this patient population, mortality may be directly related to limb function and ambulatory ability.[13] The flaps discussed in this article can help close wounds that are unamenable to primary closure and located in vulnerable areas. In the case of smaller defects (approximately 3 × 6 cm or less), a local flap is usually used when available. Larger defects or those out of reach of muscle flaps usually require a free flap. Postoperative monitoring after foot flap surgery is important in ensuring flap viability and successful outcomes. Local and free flaps are both excellent options to salvage complex wounds in the diabetic foot and show how a multidisciplinary team of podiatrists and plastic surgeons can improve outcomes in diabetic patients (**Table 3**).

REFERENCES

1. Jeffcoate WJ, Harding KG. Diabetic foot ulcers. Lancet 2003;361(9368): 1545–51.
2. Boulton AJM, Vileikyte L, Ragnarson-Tennvall G, et al. The global burden of diabetic foot disease. Lancet 2005;366(9498):1719–24.
3. Connor H. Some historical aspects of diabetic foot disease. Diabetes Metab Res Rev 2008;24(S1):S7–13.
4. Driver VR, Fabbi M, Lavery LA, et al. The costs of diabetic foot: the economic case for the limb salvage team. J Vasc Surg 2010;52(3 Suppl):17S–22S.
5. Robbins JM, Strauss G, Aron D, et al. Mortality rates and diabetic foot ulcers: is it time to communicate mortality risk to patients with diabetic foot ulceration? J Am Podiatr Med Assoc 2008;98(6):489–93.
6. Pecoraro RE, Reiber GE, Burgess EM. Pathways to diabetic limb amputation. Basis for prevention. Diabetes Care 1990;13(5):513–21.
7. Evans KK, Attinger CE, Al-Attar A, et al. The importance of limb preservation in the diabetic population. J Diabetes Complications 2011;25(4):227–31.
8. Sinkin JC, Reilly M, Cralley A, et al. Multidisciplinary approach to soft-tissue reconstruction of the diabetic Charcot foot. Plast Reconstr Surg 2015;135(2): 611–6.
9. Driver VR, Fabbi M, Lavery LA, et al. The costs of diabetic foot: the economic case for the limb salvage team. J Am Podiatr Med Assoc 2010;100(5):335–41.
10. Oh TS, Lee HS, Hong JP. Diabetic foot reconstruction using free flaps increases 5-year-survival rate. J Plast Reconstr Aesthet Surg 2013;66(2):243–50.

11. Armstrong DG, Wrobel J, Robbins JM. Guest Editorial: Are diabetes-related wounds and amputations worse than cancer? Int Wound J 2007;4(4):286–7.
12. Ducic I, Attinger CE. Foot and ankle reconstruction: pedicled muscle flaps versus free flaps and the role of diabetes. Plast Reconstr Surg 2011;128(1):173–80.
13. Engel H, Lin CH, Wei FC. Role of microsurgery in lower extremity reconstruction. Plast Reconstr Surg 2011;127(Suppl 1):228S–38S.
14. Anghel EL, DeFazio MV, Barker JC, et al. Current concepts in debridement. Plast Reconstr Surg 2016;138:82S–93S.
15. Bennett N, Choudhary S. Why climb a ladder when you can take the elevator? Plast Reconstr Surg 2000;105(6):2266–7.
16. Hollenbeck ST, Woo S, Komatsu I, et al. Longitudinal outcomes and application of the subunit principle to 165 foot and ankle free tissue transfers. Plast Reconstr Surg 2010;125(3):924–34.
17. McGregor IA, Morgan G. Axial and random pattern flaps. Br J Plast Surg 1973; 26(3):202–13.
18. Taylor GI, Palmer JH. The vascular territories (angiosomes) of the body: experimental study and clinical applications. Br J Plast Surg 1987;40(2):113–41.
19. Taylor GI, Corlett RJ, Caddy CM, et al. An anatomic review of the delay phenomenon: II. Clinical applications. Plast Reconstr Surg 1992;89(3):408–18.
20. Nakajima T, Fujino T, Adachi S. A new concept of vascular supply to the skin and classification of skin flaps according to their vascularization. Ann Plast Surg 1986; 16(1):1–19.
21. Hallock GG. Direct and indirect perforator flaps: the history and the controversy. Plast Reconstr Surg 2003;111(2):855–65.
22. Mathes SJ, Nahai F. Classification of the vascular anatomy of muscles: experimental and clinical correlation. Plast Reconstr Surg 1981;67(2):177–87.
23. Attinger CE, Evans KK, Bulan E, et al. Angiosomes of the foot and ankle and clinical implications for limb salvage: reconstruction, incisions, and revascularization. Plast Reconstr Surg 2006;117(7 Suppl):261S–93S.
24. DeFazio MV, Economides JM, Anghel EL, et al. Lower extremity free tissue transfer in the setting of thrombophilia: analysis of perioperative anticoagulation protocols and predictors of flap failure. J Reconstr Microsurg 2018. https://doi.org/10.1055/s-0038-1675145.
25. Endara M, Masden D, Goldstein J, et al. The role of chronic and perioperative glucose management in high-risk surgical closures: a case for tighter glycemic control. Plast Reconstr Surg 2013;132(4):996–1004.
26. Cho EH, Garcia RM, Pien I, et al. Vascular considerations in foot and ankle free tissue transfer: analysis of 231 free flaps. Microsurgery 2016;36(4):276–83.
27. Verhelle NA, Heymans O. How to deal with difficult microsurgical end-to-side anastomoses. Microsurgery 2005;25(3):203–8.
28. El Rifai S, Boudard J, Haiun M, et al. Tips and tricks for end-to-side anastomosis arteriotomies. Hand Surg Rehabil 2016;35:85–94.
29. DeFazio MV, Fan KL, Evans KK. Greater saphenous vein-patch interposition to facilitate flow-sparing microanastomosis of calcified arteries in the distal lower extremity. Plast Reconstr Surg, in press.
30. Eskelinen E, Kaartinen I, Kääriäinen M, et al. Successful foot salvage with microvascular flaps in diabetic patients. Scand J Surg 2014;104:103–7.
31. Lu J, DeFazio MV, Lakhiani C, et al. Limb salvage and functional outcomes following free tissue transfer for the treatment of recalcitrant diabetic foot ulcers. J Reconstr Microsurg 2019;35(2):117–23.

32. Hanasono MM, Skoracki RJ, Yu P. A prospective study of donor-site morbidity after anterolateral thigh fasciocutaneous and myocutaneous free flap harvest in 220 patients. Plast Reconstr Surg 2010;125(1):209–14.
33. Ger R. The operative treatment of the advanced stasis ulcer: a preliminary communication. Am J Surg 1966;111:659–63.
34. Ger R. The management of pre-tibial skin loss. Surgery 1968;63:757–63.
35. Ger R. Operative treatment of the advanced stasis ulcer using muscle transposition. Am J Surg 1970;120:376–80.
36. Ger R. The technique of muscle transposition and the operative treatment of traumatic and ulcerative lesions of the leg. J Trauma 1971;11:502–10.
37. Attinger CE, Ducic I, Cooper P, et al. The role of intrinsic muscle flaps of the foot for bone coverage in foot and anke defects in diabetic and nondiabetic patients. Plast Reconstr Surg 2002;110:1047–54.
38. Ger R. Newer concepts in the surgical management of lesions of the foot in the patient with diabetes. Surg Gynecol Obstet 1984;158:213–5.
39. Yoshimura Y, Nakajima T, Kami T. Distally based abductor digiti minimi muscle flap. Ann Plast Surg 1985;14:375–7.
40. Neale HW, Stern PJ, Kreilein JG, et al. Complications of muscle-flap transposition for traumatic defects of the leg. Plast Reconstr Surg 1983;72(4):512–7.
41. Serafin D, Georgiade NG, Smith DH. Comparison of free flaps with pedicled flaps for coverage of defects of the leg or foot. Plast Reconstr Surg 1977;59:492–9.
42. Wei FC, Mardini S. Flaps and reconstructive surgery. 2nd edition. New York: Elsevier; 2017.
43. Thorne CH, editor. Grabb and Smith's plastic surgery. 7th edition. Philadelphia: Wolters Kluwer; 2014.
44. Willy C, Agarwal A, Andersen CA, et al. Closed incision negative pressure therapy: international multidisciplinary consensus recommendations. Int Wound J 2017;14(2):385–98.

Bone Reconstruction in the Diabetic Foot

Brett C. Chatman, DPM, AACFAS*, Virginia E. Parks, DPM, AACFAS

KEYWORDS

- Surgical reconstruction • Diabetic foot • Bone reconstruction • Deformity correction

KEY POINTS

- This article discusses preventive and prophylactic surgical bone reconstruction procedures to reduce osseous deformity, minimize pre-ulcerative lesions and increase limb salvage rates in the compromised patient with diabetes.
- Focus is on the statistical evidence as to why preventive surgical intervention is of the utmost importance and should be considered when performing a diabetic foot risk evaluation.
- Surgical bone correction in patients with preexisting wounds to increase wound healing and prevent possible infection with amputation is also addressed.

INTRODUCTION

When performing a diabetic foot evaluation for patients with preulcerative lesions or preexisting wounds, it is imperative to address surgical bone reconstructive procedures of the foot and ankle. Lower extremity foot and ankle ulcerations, wounds, infections, and amputations have increased dramatically with the increased prevalence of diabetes in our society. Approximately 1% to 4% of patients with diabetes develop a new foot ulceration every year.[1,2] In evaluating lower extremity disease (LED) in the United States, it has been shown that the incidence of LED is twice as high among individuals with diabetes than in those without diabetes.[3] Van Battum and colleagues[4] reported that among patients with diabetes there is a 25% lifetime risk of developing a foot ulceration, of which the majority will need surgical intervention within 4 years of the initial diagnosis. Large and small musculoskeletal deformities can lead to increased plantar pressures as well as increased friction, and are the primary cause of preulcerative lesions or diabetic foot ulcers. Reiber and associates[5,6] showed that foot deformity associated with neuropathy and minor trauma accounted for more than 63% of all foot ulcers. If the aim is to correct the potential pathologic

Disclosures: The authors have nothing to disclose.
Department of Surgery, Division of Plastic and Reconstructive Surgery, Hospital of the University of Pennsylvania, 3400 Civic Center Boulevard, Philadelphia, PA 19104, USA
* Corresponding author.
E-mail address: Brett.Chatman@uphs.upenn.edu

etiology with preventive surgical intervention, the probability that a patient will develop a preulcerative lesion, ulceration, or potential infection is decreased. The aim of this article is to outline specific bony deformities, analyze how they are at risk for developing lesions, and discuss surgical bone reconstructive procedures for deformity correction.

THE FACTS

When evaluating patients with diabetes who present to the office with an at-risk foot, it is important for the foot and ankle surgeon to have a variety of surgical techniques in the armamentarium for the prevention of ulceration. If the foot and ankle surgeon lays primary focus on the correction of the etiology of a wound or prevention of wound occurrence, one can dramatically decrease the amount of amputations that happen each year and increase the number of limbs salvaged. Foot ulcerations are the initial inciting event in more than 85% of major amputations that are performed on patients with diabetes.[7] Apelqvist and associates[8] reported that 70% of patients with diabetic foot ulcers will suffer recurrence within 5 years. In 2017, this same group performed a similar study and noted that 42% of their patient population developed a recurrent foot ulcer.[9] In a separate study in 2018, Khalifa[10] reported that 61.3% of patients had recurrent foot ulcers within a 2-year study period. Furthermore, several studies have reported on the overall morbidity and mortality of patients who initially present with a diabetic foot ulcer, and all results have been generally poor.[11–15] The Centers for Disease Control and Prevention (CDC) reported that in patients with diabetes there are approximately 73,000 nontraumatic lower-limb amputations performed annually with more than 85% of those amputations being preceded by a foot ulcer.[16]

Ulcerations have a complex multifactorial etiology, with several causative factors being well described. Excessive plantar pressure from limited joint mobility and foot deformities was shown to be a major causative factor of ulceration, with peripheral neuropathy being present in more than 50% of patients.[17] The presence of peripheral arterial disease (PAD) has also been shown to be a major causative factor in the diabetic population, leading to neuroischemic ulceration. Boulton and colleagues[18] showed that PAD and neuropathy are involved in approximately 45% of diabetic foot ulcers. Neuropathy, vascular disease, and poor glycemic control, as well as other medical comorbidities, all significantly contribute to increased risk of foot ulceration and postoperative complications after surgical intervention. For these reasons, the key to successful bone reconstruction in the patient with diabetes is a multidisciplinary team approach with medical and surgical optimization. Early correction of deformity before disease progression can reduce the risk of pressure-induced ulcers, subsequent infection, and even limb loss by creating a more biomechanically favorable foot. In the authors' opinion, prevention of ulceration by management of causative factors is imperative to prevent recurrence of the wound, wound infection, and subsequent amputation, thereby decreasing associated morbidity and mortality.

BONE RECONSTRUCTION

When deciding to proceed with elective or prophylactic surgery, there should be no active infection. If there is an active infection, surgical debridement with removal of all nonviable soft tissue and bone should be performed before any definitive procedure. If there is diagnosed osteomyelitis, surgical removal of the affected bone should be prioritized. Throughout this article, different surgical options for bone reconstruction of the diabetic foot are reviewed. These procedures focus on prevention of recurrence of ulcerations for limb salvage but do not address Charcot reconstruction of the lower extremity, which will be addressed separately. The choice of surgical intervention should ultimately be patient specific and depend on the cause of the wound. A multidisciplinary team approach should be used for medical optimization before surgical intervention in the case of nonurgent or elective surgical correction.

Elective Surgery for Digital Deformities

Khalifa[10] reported that 33% of recurrent ulcers are located in the forefoot. Contracture deformities of the lesser digits such as hammertoes, claw toes, and mallet toes are very common in both the diabetic and nondiabetic populations. In those patients without diabetes, the greatest concerns are typically pain with shoe wear caused by friction on the prominent dorsal aspect of the contracted joint or dissatisfaction with appearance. Although the diabetic patient without neuropathy may share similar concerns, the patient with neuropathy is significantly less likely to experience pain attributable to friction and pressure with shoe wear. Any osseous prominence or area of focal increased pressure becomes at increased risk for ulceration. In particular, rigidly contracted hammertoes will experience increased pressure and friction on the dorsal proximal interphalangeal joint and distal tip of the digit, as shown in **Fig. 1**. Claw toe deformities, with contracture of both the proximal interphalangeal joint (PIPJ) and distal interphalangeal joint (DIPJ), will experience increased pressure to the dorsal aspect of both joints as well as the distal tip of the digit. Mallet toes demonstrate contracture primarily at the DIPJ and will have pressure dorsal to the DIPJ as well as the distal tip of the toe. Because the soft-tissue coverage dorsal to these joint tends to be somewhat thin, especially with skin atrophy in patients with diabetes and peripheral vascular disease, a dorsal ulcer on a contracted interphalangeal joint can quickly progress to the level of the extensor tendon, joint capsule, and joint. In turn this can quickly progress to osteomyelitis or infection that travels along the tendon sheath. Infected ulcers on the tip of the contracted toe that probe to bone on the distal phalanx can progress to infection that travels proximally along either the flexor or extensor tendon sheath. Therefore, if the patient with digital contracture has a well-controlled hemoglobin A1c with adequate perfusion, surgical correction of the deformity should be considered to prevent ulcerations that can easily lead to digital soft-tissue and bone infections (see **Fig. 1**).

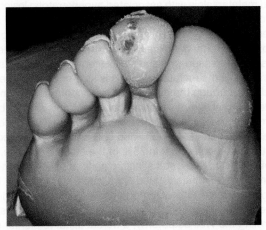

Fig. 1. Increased plantar pressure secondary to a hammertoe deformity causing an ulceration at the distal tip of the second digit.

When addressing deformities of the lesser digits, it is important to determine whether the etiology of the hammertoe, claw toe, or mallet toe is flexible, semirigid, or rigid. Rigid contracture deformities require correction of the structural deformity with an osseous surgical procedure to reduce the deformity, decrease bony prominences, and more evenly disperse pressures throughout the digit. If the deformity is flexible, soft-tissue release of the joint contracture is recommended and can preserve the structural stability of the toe. If the deformity is located at the DIPJ with pressure at the distal tip of the digit, as seen in a mallet toe, a flexor tenotomy at the DIPJ can reduce the contracture and alleviate plantar pressure. If the deformity is located at the DIPJ and PIPJ, a flexor tenotomy at the PIPJ should be performed to release both the long and the short flexors.[19]

If the deformity is isolated to a single digit, joint arthroplasty or arthrodesis can be considered; however, one should take into consideration that an aggressive arthroplasty does destabilize the digit and could lead to further deformity. If multiple digital procedures are required, the interphalangeal joint arthrodesis is recommended to convert the digit to a rigid lever arm and allow stability at the metatarsophalangeal joint (MPJ). With both procedures, a dorsolinear incision or 2 transverse semielliptical incisions can be created over the joint. If a lesion is present, all tissue incorporating the lesion down to the level of the extensor tendon is removed. The extensor tendon is then transected transversely to allow for optimal visualization of the desired joints. Transverse osteotomies of the desired joints are then performed with pin fixation for stabilization.

Special consideration should be given to the reduction of the hammertoe deformity of the fifth digit because hyperkeratotic lesions of the fifth digit can lead to complicated wounds in the insensate foot. Fifth-digit deformities, as well as tight-fitting shoes, typically lead to a heloma durum on the dorsolateral aspect of the DIPJ, as shown in **Figs. 2** and **3**. Surgical planning should take into consideration the specific location of the preulcerative lesion. If the underlying cause is a dorsal exostosis or accessory bone, a simple exosectomy can be performed with a derotational skin plasty. Partial versus complete arthroplasties should be considered when addressing the pressure keratosis (see **Figs. 2** and **3**).

Elective Surgery for Lesser Metatarsal Head Deformities

Pressure-induced metatarsalgia with associated hyperkeratotic lesions requires surgical intervention for complete resolution. Surgical options consist of an osteotomy of the metatarsal versus a condylectomy.[20] If the lesion is due to a sagittal plane deformity, a dorsiflexory osteotomy is typically performed. If excessive length of a metatarsal is the cause of increased pressure, an osteotomy should also be performed to correct the parabola of the metatarsals. This is key for appropriate weight distribution during ambulation through the gait cycle. Prominent plantar condyles can cause high areas of plantar pressure. A plantar condylectomy should be performed to remove the deforming force and should also be considered if the patient is not an ideal candidate for internal fixation. Vandeputte and colleagues[21] published a study looking at the Weil osteotomy and noted that in 75% of the studied patients, there was complete resolution of the callus with a statistically significant decrease in plantar pressure load under the involved metatarsal head. In a separate study by Khalafi and colleagues,[22] after performing a Weil osteotomy there was a 36% reduction of plantar pressure in the neutral position and a 65% reduction of plantar pressure during heel rise. When performing the Weil osteotomy, a dorsal distal to plantar proximal osteotomy is made at a 45° angle at the level of the surgical neck typically fixated with a 2.0 cortical screw.[23,24] According to Guirini,[25] a dorsal to plantar V-shaped osteotomy

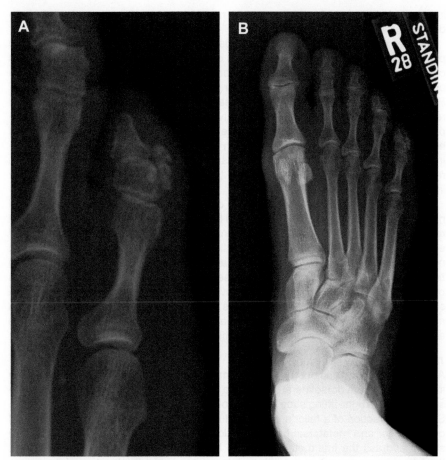

Fig. 2. (*A*, *B*) Preoperative radiograph of a fifth-digit osteophyte causing a preulcerative lesion in a patient with diabetes.

with the apex pointing distally allows for adequate relief of the plantar pressures overlying the ulceration. Fixation is performed with a 0.045 Kirschner wire and the patient is kept non–weight bearing for 4 to 6 weeks. One should take into consideration the potential risk of transfer lesions when performing lesser metatarsal osteotomies. Again, it

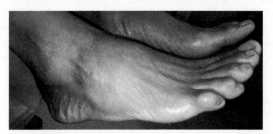

Fig. 3. Clinical photo correlating to the radiographs in **Fig. 1** of fifth-digit osteophyte causing a preulcerative lesion in a patient with diabetes.

is extremely important for the surgeon to maintain a normal metatarsal parabola to decrease the risk of transfer lesions.

Another option for treatment of neuropathic diabetic foot ulcers located on the plantar surface of the metatarsal heads is complete metatarsal head resection. It is often thought that metatarsal head resection should only be used in the case of osteomyelitis, owing to the high rate of transfer lesions. In a 2017 article in the *Journal of Foot and Ankle Surgery*, Motamedi and Ansari[26] showed that surgical metatarsal head resection, when compared with conservative medical management for these neuropathic plantar ulcerations, showed complete superiority with an increase in wound healing and a lower long-term complication rate. It should be noted that when resecting a metatarsal head, the base of the associated proximal phalanx should also be resected because it is contiguous with the metatarsal head and is most likely involved.[25]

When the metatarsal parabola has been disrupted or there are noted to be several nonhealing ulcerations, multiple metatarsal head resections or a pan-metatarsal head resection may be indicated. In 2012, Armstrong and coworkers[27] looked at the clinical efficacy of the pan-metatarsal head resection as a curative procedure in those with neuropathic forefoot wounds and noted that they are associated with shorter healing times and have a lower morbidity than conservative management. This procedure can be performed through a single plantar transverse incision made in the relaxed skin tension lines directly over the metatarsal heads or via multiple dorsal incisions.[28] With this approach, weight bearing becomes proximal to the incision once the metatarsal heads are removed and pressure-related problems are alleviated.[28]

Tailor's bunion

A tailor's bunion, or bunionette, is a deformity of the fifth metatarsal head leading to increased pressure dorsolateral or lateral to the metatarsal head. This increased pressure along with tight-fitting shoe wear can often lead to ulceration, as shown in **Fig. 4**. Surgical correction of a tailor's bunion includes condylectomies, distal and proximal osteotomies, and metatarsal head resection. When addressing the deformity, one should address the intermetatarsal angle between the fourth and fifth metatarsal, the lateral bowing angle of the fifth metatarsal head, and the location of the lesion. If the deformity is mild to moderate, a condylectomy may be performed. Incision is placed dorsolateral to the fifth metatarsal. After careful dissection and exposure, approximately one-third to one-fourth of the lateral metatarsal head is removed. Distal osteotomies typically involve a chevron osteotomy with a transposition of the distal fragment. Proximal osteotomies are used when the deformity is too severe for a distal osteotomy, but are rarely indicated. As previously mentioned, if the deformity of the metatarsal head is severe enough, or there is presence of a recurring ulceration, metatarsal head resection is a valuable procedure in the neuropathic patient. The osteotomy is performed in a dorsal-distal-lateral to plantar-proximal-medial orientation. Armstrong and colleagues[29] performed a study looking at the efficacy of the fifth metatarsal head resection for treatment of chronic diabetic foot ulceration, and noted that patients healed significantly faster and were much less likely to reulcerate with resection in comparison with those who underwent conservative management (see **Fig. 4**).

Elective Surgery for First-Ray Deformities

Hallux

The location of the ulceration on the lower extremity tells a unique story about the underlying etiology. Khalifa[10] reported that 24.6% of recurrent ulcerations were located

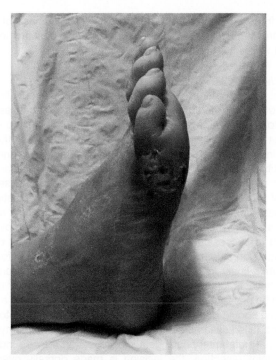

Fig. 4. Clinical photo of a lateral fifth metatarsal head wound secondary to a tailor's bunion and tight-fitting shoe wear.

on the hallux. The first ray is often seen as a common location for ulceration to occur, as plantar pressures are peaked under the hallux in comparison with the rest of the foot during the gait cycle.[30] Limited range of motion at the first MPJ can lead to excessive plantar pressure and ulceration during ambulation. Ulcerations of the hallux primarily occur plantar-medial or directly plantar to the interphalangeal joint. High areas of plantar pressure can be caused by an interphalangeal joint (IPJ) sesamoid, enlarged condyles of the phalanx, or hyperextension of the IPJ compensating secondary to hallux limitus or rigidus. In cases where there is adequate range of motion of the metatarsal phalangeal joint and the underlying problem is an enlarged condyle or an IPJ sesamoid, removal of the sesamoid or excision of the proximal phalanx head will alleviate the plantar pressure causing the ulceration. In cases of decreased dorsiflexion of the hallux on the metatarsal head, as seen in hallux rigidus/limitus, addressing the MPJ is necessary. In these situations one may perform an arthroplasty of the base of the proximal phalanx in an effort to increase the range of motion of the MPJ. Armstrong and colleagues[31] published a study with results suggesting that the resection arthroplasty is an effective procedure to treat plantar hallux wounds when compared with nonsurgical therapy, whereby patients healed significantly faster and had fewer recurrent ulcers.

The Keller arthroplasty is also indicated when there is extensive degeneration of the first MPJ.[32] A dorsomedial linear incision is made mid-diaphysis of the first metatarsal extending to just shy of the IPJ. Adequate exposure is obtained, exposing the first metatarsal head and base of the proximal phalanx. Bonney and Macnab[33] reported that when creating the osteotomy, one-third to one-half was the optimal amount of bone resection from the proximal phalanx to allow for purchase of the hallux. If a plantar ulcer is present the surgeon may consider creating a plantar incision, excising the ulcer in total with a full-thickness primary closure.[25]

First metatarsal head

Moving proximal along the first ray, ulcerations frequently occur directly plantar or plantar-medial to the first metatarsal head. There are several causes for ulcerations directly plantar to the first metatarsal head, and one should take into account the position of the first metatarsal when considering the pathology of these ulcerations (**Fig. 5**). If the first metatarsal is *not* noted to be plantarflexed, one may consider removal of the tibial sesamoid, fibular sesamoid, or both. The sesamoids articulate directly with the plantar surface of the first metatarsal head and serve to improve the efficiency of the flexor hallucis longus tendon. When ambulating through the gait cycle, the sesamoids migrate distally and can act as a distinct area of pressure directly under the plantar metatarsal head, causing ulceration. Removal of these sesamoids can lead to successful healing of the ulcer.[34,35] The most commonly used incision is a medial longitudinal incision plantar to a standard bunion incision. With careful dissection, a linear longitudinal capsular incision is made dorsal to the fibers of the abductor hallucis tendon and the sesamoids are identified.[36] If the first metatarsal is noted to be plantarflexed, a sesamoidectomy is considered a relative contraindication and one should consider a dorsiflexory metatarsal osteotomy. If a patient reulcerates after a failed sesamoidectomy, or there is noted osteomyelitis of the first metatarsal head, a metatarsal phalangeal joint resection may be indicated.[32] When performing this joint resection, the incision is made dorsally over the first MPJ directly down to bone, obtaining adequate exposure of the proximal phalanx base and first metatarsal head. It is imperative to perform a smooth osteotomy of the metatarsal head to not allow for any osseous prominences that could act as a source of pressure.

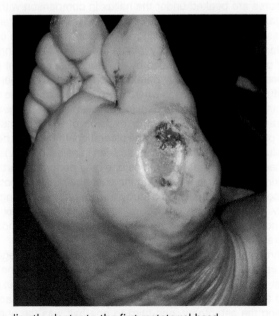

Fig. 5. Ulceration directly plantar to the first metatarsal head.

Bunion Deformity

Hallux abducto valgus (HAV) is a deformity of the first metatarsal and has a multifactorial etiology. Typically, patients present with a dorsal or dorsomedial exostosis that ranges in size based on the severity of the deformity present. A large exostosis can be a point of ulceration in the at-risk foot (**Fig. 6**). When evaluating all patients, baseline radiographs are appropriate to determine the severity of the deformity as mild, moderate, or severe. In patients with diabetes, ulceration can occur from shearing forces from tight-fitting shoes rubbing against the exostosis. Nonoperative preventive treatment consists of the patient being fit for a custom molded orthotic from a specialized orthotist to offload any bony prominences with accommodative inserts and shoe gear that will not cause rubbing of the bunion. Operative management of deformity correction to prevent potential wound breakdown should be addressed with each patient, and careful patient selection should be performed. If the intermetatarsal angle is within normal limits or is noted to be mild, a silver bunionectomy can be performed, which will include removal of the exostosis and a possible capsulotomy to obtain appropriate alignment and position of the sesamoids. Distal metaphyseal osteotomies are the most common correction of the HAV deformity and are normally used for mild to moderate intermetatarsal angles. A dorsomedial incision extending from the midshaft of the metatarsal to just proximal to the hallux IPJ with a careful layered dissection is performed. Next, a plantar lateral soft-tissue contracture release is performed along exposure of the metatarsal head as needed. After adequate resection of the dorsomedial eminence, an osteotomy of the metatarsal head can be performed and fixated based on the procedure of choice as selected by the surgeon. Proximal metatarsal osteotomies are indicated if the first ray is noted to be rigid with moderate to severe intermetatarsal angle or if the first metatarsal is noted to be elevated and hypermobile. Several different types of procedures have been described for proximal metatarsal osteotomies. Incision placement normally extends from the first metatarsal-cuneiform joint to the proximal phalanx of the hallux.[37] After the MPJ is released and the medial eminence is excised, an osteotomy at the base of the first metatarsal can be performed based on the procedure of choice by the surgeon.

Tendoachilles Lengthening

Although this article covers bone reconstruction in the diabetic foot, the authors considered it necessary to briefly discuss the importance of the tendoachilles-lengthening procedure. Patients who have diabetes are often noted to have contracture of the gastrocnemius-soleus muscle complex and Achilles tendon. A high blood glucose over a long period of time can lead to enzymatic glycosylation of the Achilles tendon, causing it to become tight and contracted. When the Achilles tendon becomes contracted and tight, it causes increased plantar forefoot pressures and may be a primary reason for reulceration or failure of the surgical procedure if not addressed. Armstrong and colleagues[38] published a study showing that a

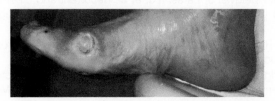

Fig. 6. Ulceration medial to the first metatarsal head secondary to HAV deformity.

percutaneous tendoachilles lengthening significantly reduced peak pressures on the forefoot and should be used for diabetic patients who are at high risk for ulceration of the foot. The rate of ulcer recurrence was lower following Achilles tendon lengthening or gastrocnemius recession procedures in comparison with other treatment options alone.[39]

SUMMARY

Bone reconstruction of the diabetic foot is a complex topic that needs to be considered and addressed with each individual patient. It is important to analyze the etiology of any deformity in the at-risk foot by performing a thorough biomechanical evaluation. This is of the utmost importance while performing a diabetic foot risk evaluation to help the surgeon address any potential areas of concern in the diabetic foot. Deformity identification and surgical bone reconstruction can help prevent the patient from developing an ulceration or infection, and may potentially save their limb. Limb salvage is truly a multidisciplinary team approach; with careful patient selection, medical optimization, appropriate blood flow evaluation/revascularization, and careful surgical biomechanical planning, clinicians can truly help to save limbs and save lives.

REFERENCES

1. Wu S, Driver V, Wrobel J, et al. Foot ulcers in the diabetic patient, prevention and treatment. Vasc Health Risk Manag 2007;3(1):65–76.
2. Ignatiadis II, Tsiampa VA, Papalois AE. A systematic approach to the failed plastic surgical reconstruction of the diabetic foot. Diabet Foot Ankle 2011;2(1):6435.
3. Ylitalo KR, Sowers M, Heeringa S. Peripheral vascular disease and peripheral neuropathy in individuals with cardiometabolic clustering and obesity: National Health and Nutrition Examination Survey 2001-2004. Diabetes Care 2011;34(7): 1642–7.
4. van Battum P, Schaper N, Prompers L, et al. Differences in minor amputation rate in diabetic foot disease throughout Europe are in part explained by differences in disease severity at presentation. Diabet Med 2011;28:199–205.
5. Gregg EW, Sorlie P, Paulose-Ram R, et al. Prevalence of lower-extremity disease in the US adult population ≥40 years of age with an without diabetes: 1999-2000 national health and nutrition examination survey. Diabetes Care 2004;27(7): 1591–7.
6. Pitcher JM, Wooden WA. Plastic surgical reconstruction of the diabetic foot. In: Bowker JH, Pfeifer MA, editors. Levin and O'Neal's the diabetic foot. Maryland Heights (MO): Mosby Elsevier; 2008. p. 443–60.
7. Brownrigg JR, Apelqvist J, Bakker K, et al. Evidence-based management of PAD & the diabetic foot. Eur J Vasc Endovasc Surg 2013;45(6):673–81.
8. Apelqvist J, Larsson J, Agardh CD. Long-term prognosis for diabetic patients with foot ulcers. J Intern Med 1993;233(6):485–91.
9. Örneholm H, Apelqvist J, Larsson J, et al. Recurrent and other new foot ulcers after healed plantar forefoot diabetic ulcer. Wound Repair Regen 2017;25(2): 309–15.
10. Khalifa WA. Risk factors for diabetic foot ulcer recurrence: a prospective 2-year follow-up study in Egypt. Foot (Edinb) 2018;35:11–5.
11. Ndosi M, Wright-Hughes A, Brown S, et al. Prognosis of the infected diabetic foot ulcer: a 12-month prospective observational study. Diabet Med 2017;35(1): 78–88.

12. Singh N, Armstrong DG, Lipsky BA. Preventing foot ulcers in patients with diabetes. JAMA 2005;293(2):217.
13. American Diabetes Association. Fast facts: data and statistics about diabetes. Arlington (VA): American Diabetes Association; 2015.
14. Clayton W, Elasy TA. A review of the pathophysiology, classification, and treatment of foot ulcers in diabetic patients. Clin Diabetes 2009;27(2):52–8.
15. Humphers JM, Shibuya N, Fluhman BL, et al. The impact of glycosylated hemoglobin and diabetes mellitus on wound-healing complications and infection after foot and ankle surgery. J Am Podiatr Med Assoc 2014;104(4):320–9.
16. Centers for Disease Control and Prevention. National diabetes statistics report: estimates of diabetes and its burden in the United States, 2014. Atlanta (GA): US Department of Health and Human Services; 2014.
17. Viswanathan V, Snehalatha C, Sivagami M, et al. Association of limited joint mobility and high plantar pressure in diabetic foot ulceration in Asian Indians. Diabetes Res Clin Pract 2003;60(1):57–61.
18. Boulton AJ, Kirsner RS, Vileikyte L. Clinical practice. "Neuropathic diabetic foot ulcers. N Engl J Med 2004;351:48–55.
19. Boberg JS, Willis JJ. Lesser digital deformities: etiology, procedural selection, and arthroplasty. In: Southerland JT, Boberg JS, Downey MS, et al, editors. McGlamry's comprehensive textbook of foot and ankle surgery. Philadelphia (PA): Wolters Kluwer/Lippincott Williams & Wilkins Health; 2013. p. 124–8.
20. Southerland JT, Boberg JS, Downey MS, et al, editors. McGlamry's comprehensive textbook of foot and ankle surgery. Philadelphia (PA): Wolters Kluwer/Lippincott Williams & Wilkins Health; 2013.
21. Vandeputte G, Dereymaeker G, Steenwerckx A, et al. The Weil osteotomy of the lesser metatarsals: a clinical and pedobarographic follow-up study. Foot Ankle Int 2000;21(5):370–4.
22. Khalafi A, Landsman AS, Lautenschlager EP, et al. Plantar forefoot pressure changes after second metatarsal neck osteotomy. Foot Ankle Int 2005;26(7):550–5.
23. Huerta JP, Lorente CA, Carmona FJC. The Weil osteotomy: a comprehensive review. Revista Española De Podología 2017;28(2):e38–51.
24. Hobizal KB, Wukich DK. Diabetic foot infections: current concept review. Diabet Foot Ankle 2012. https://doi.org/10.3402/dfa.v3i0.18409.
25. Giurini J. The diabetic foot: medical and surgical management. Springer International; 2018.
26. Kalantar Motamedi A, Ansari M. Comparison of metatarsal head resection versus conservative care in treatment of neuropathic diabetic foot ulcers. J Foot Ankle Surg 2017;56(3):428–33.
27. Armstrong DG, Fiorito JL, Leykum BJ, et al. Clinical efficacy of the Pan metatarsal head resection as a curative procedure in patients with diabetes mellitus and neuropathic forefoot wounds. Foot Ankle Spec 2012;5(4):235–40.
28. Miller MJ, Masadeh SB. Plantar foot surgery. In: Southerland JT, Boberg JS, Downey MS, et al, editors. McGlamry's comprehensive textbook of foot and ankle surgery. Philadelphia (PA): Wolters Kluwer/Lippincott Williams & Wilkins Health; 2013. p. 513–24.
29. Armstrong DG, Rosales MA, Gashi A. Efficacy of fifth metatarsal head resection for treatment of chronic diabetic foot ulceration. J Am Podiatr Med Assoc 2005; 95(4):353–6.
30. Nandikolla VK, Bochen R, Meza S, et al. Experimental gait analysis to study stress distribution of the human foot. J Med Eng 2017;2017:1–13.

31. Armstrong DG, Lavery LA, Vazquez JR, et al. Clinical efficacy of the first metatar-sophalangeal joint arthroplasty as a curative procedure for hallux interphalangeal joint wounds in patients with diabetes. Diabetes Care 2003;26(12):3284–7.
32. Frykberg RG, Bevilacqua NJ, Habershaw G. Surgical off-loading of the diabetic foot. J Vasc Surg 2010;52(3):44S–58S.
33. Bonney G, Macnab I. Hallux valgus and hallux rigidus; a critical survey of operative results. J Bone Joint Surg Br 1952;34-B(3):366–85.
34. Giurini JM, Chrzan JS, Gibbons GW, et al. Sesamoidectomy for the treatment of chronic neuropathic ulcerations. J Am Podiatr Med Assoc 1991;81(4):167–73.
35. Tamir E, Tamir J, Beer Y, et al. Resection arthroplasty for resistant ulcers underlying the hallux in insensate diabetics. Foot Ankle Int 2015;36(8):969–75.
36. Lee S. Technique of isolated tibial sesamoidectomy. Techniques in Foot & Ankle Surgery 2004;3(2):85–90.
37. Mothershed RE. Proximal osteotomies of the first metataral. In: Southerland JT, Boberg JS, Downey MS, et al, editors. McGlamry's comprehensive textbook of foot and ankle surgery. Philadelphia (PA): Wolters Kluwer/Lippincott Williams & Wilkins Health; 2013. p. 290–301.
38. Armstrong DG, Stacpoole-Shea S, Nguyen H, et al. Lengthening of the Achilles tendon in diabetic patients who are at high risk for ulceration of the foot. J Bone Joint Surg Am 1999;81(4):535–8.
39. Dallimore SM, Kaminski MR. Tendon lengthening and fascia release for healing and preventing diabetic foot ulcers: a systematic review and meta-analysis. J Foot Ankle Res 2015;8:33.

Optimizing Results in Diabetic Charcot Reconstruction

Katherine M. Raspovic, DPM*, George T. Liu, DPM,
Trapper Lalli, MD, Michael Van Pelt, DPM, Dane K. Wukich, MD

KEYWORDS

- Charcot neuroarthropathy • Charcot reconstruction • Surgical optimization
- Preoperative evaluation • Intraoperative techniques • Diabetic Charcot patient

KEY POINTS

- This first portion of this article reviews the preoperative evaluation and work-up of the diabetic Charcot patient. The goal is to help surgeons identify modifiable factors that, if improved, may help optimize postoperative outcomes.
- The second portion of this article reviews intraoperative techniques to help optimize postoperative outcomes.
- Objective measures of patient outcomes will become increasingly important with the transition to value-based care.

INTRODUCTION

Reconstruction of the diabetic Charcot foot can be a challenge even for experienced surgeons. In addition to peripheral neuropathy and diabetes mellitus (DM), patients often present with additional comorbidities, including peripheral arterial disease, end-stage renal disease, anemia, and coronary artery disease, all of which can have an impact on the postoperative outcome. Patient selection, preoperative medical optimization, and a well-planned surgical intervention are key and may help reduce perioperative complications. There are nonmodifiable factors that a surgeon cannot control, such as neuropathy, for example, that have been shown to increase risk for postoperative complications.[1] Modifiable risk factors should be addressed prior to embarking on Charcot reconstruction, whenever possible. The aim of this review is to discuss the key elements of the preoperative medical optimization, surgical

Disclosures: The authors have nothing to disclose.
Department of Orthopaedic Surgery, University of Texas Southwestern Medical Center, 1801 Inwood Road, Dallas, TX 75390, USA
* Corresponding author.
E-mail address: Katherine.Raspovic@utsouthwestern.edu

planning, surgical reconstruction, and postoperative care to optimize the potential for a successful outcome.

PART 1: PREOPERATIVE EVALUATION AND PLANNING
History and Examination

A comprehensive history and examination are critical when deciding if a patient requires Charcot neuroarthropathy (CN) reconstruction. The history of present illness should detail recent or remote injury, character, and duration of symptoms and treatment thus far. Patients may not recall any precipitating trauma, be it major or minor. Often, patients relate a recent change in activity, such as a recent vacation requiring a lot of walking and touring or an increase in yard work. In many patients, unexplained swelling is a presenting symptom that has an impact on the ability to wear shoes. Despite the presence of neuropathy, some patients may have pain and that should be quantified using the visual analog scale (0–10). Key findings in the review of systems include any recent constitutional symptoms (fever or chills), lower extremity claudication or rest pain, history of ulceration or infection, and current or remote foot-related hospitalization. Previous foot or ankle surgery should be documented.

The past medical history and problem list should document the presence or absence of important risk factors that are associated with perioperative complications (cardiovascular, respiratory, and renal). Diabetes history should include duration of DM, method of glycemic control (oral, diet, or insulin), most recent hemoglobin A_{1C} (HbA$_{1C}$), fasting blood glucose, ulceration history (even if there is not a current ulcer), history of foot infection/hospitalization, previous vascular interventions, cardiac history, use of tobacco products, type of employment, presence and extent of renal disease, use of anticoagulation, history of deep venous thrombosis, and previous amputations. Evaluation of a patient's current shoes, inserts, and bracing should be included. In addition to the foot and ankle evaluation, a comprehensive preoperative history and physical examination should be performed by an appropriate medical consultant. The utilization of subspecialty consultants is encouraged (vascular, endocrine, renal, cardiology, and so forth).

The clinical examination should include an assessment of vascular (palpation of pedal and popliteal pulses and presence of edema), sensory (monofilament, vibratory sensation, and Achilles reflexes), dermatologic (presence or absence of ulcer and or preulcerative lesions), and musculoskeletal (location and extent of CN deformity) systems. The CN foot should be assessed for tendon/soft tissue contracture due to long-standing deformity. Muscle and tendon strength should be evaluated (ie overpowering or weakness). Osseous deformity/alignment (varus, valgus, or plantar collapse) should be assessed, when a patient is weight bearing, if possible. In general, indications for CN surgical intervention are deformity with an impending ulceration, recurrent ulceration, nonhealing ulceration, progressively worsening deformity, and an unstable foot/ankle that is not amenable to bracing. Although patients with CN have neuropathy, some patients may complain of acute or worsening pain that interferes with activities of daily living.

Preoperative Laboratory Tests and Testing: Noninvasive Arterial Studies

(Fig. 1) Even in the setting of palpable pedal pulses, the authors suggest obtaining noninvasive arterial studies, to include ankle-brachial indices (ABI), toe-brachial indices (TBI), and toe pressure measurements. Abnormal findings should prompt referral to a consultant experienced in revascularization prior to elective surgery. Depending on the geography, this may include a vascular surgeon, interventional

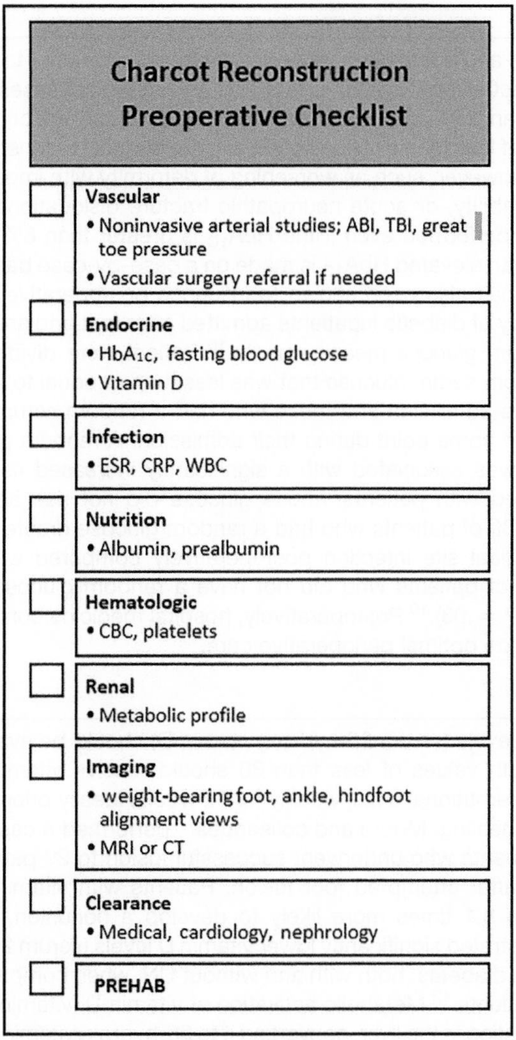

Charcot Reconstruction Preoperative Checklist

☐ **Vascular**
  - Noninvasive arterial studies; ABI, TBI, great toe pressure
  - Vascular surgery referral if needed

☐ **Endocrine**
  - HbA1c, fasting blood glucose
  - Vitamin D

☐ **Infection**
  - ESR, CRP, WBC

☐ **Nutrition**
  - Albumin, prealbumin

☐ **Hematologic**
  - CBC, platelets

☐ **Renal**
  - Metabolic profile

☐ **Imaging**
  - weight-bearing foot, ankle, hindfoot alignment views
  - MRI or CT

☐ **Clearance**
  - Medical, cardiology, nephrology

☐ **PREHAB**

Fig. 1. Charcot reconstruction preoperative checklist: key studies, laboratory tests, and medical referrals that should be obtained prior to surgical intervention. WBC, white blood cell count. (*Courtesy of* UT Southwestern Medical Center, Dallas, TX.)

cardiologist, or interventional radiologist. Gregg and colleagues[2] estimated the prevalence of peripheral artery disease (PAD) in patients with DM over the age of 40 to be approximately 10%. Wukich and colleagues[3] retrospectively evaluated a group of 85 patients with CN and DM and compared this cohort a group of 126 patients with diabetic foot ulceration (DFU) and no CN. Patients with DFU were significantly more likely to have PAD compared to patients with CN. Although critical limb ischemia is relatively rare in patients with CN, PAD was identified in approximately 40% of patients. It is important to recognize that patients with DM are more likely to have falsely elevated ABIs due to medial artery calcinosis. Because the much smaller arteries of the toe are less affected by this, an abnormal TBI is more helpful to diagnose PAD.[4–6] A great toe pressure of 55 mm Hg may be adequate for wound healing.[7–9]

Glycemic Control

Optimal long-term and short-term glycemic control is paramount to reducing complications. A prospective study of 2000 foot and ankle surgical cases reported that an HbA_{1C} greater than 8% was associated with surgical site infection.[1] The authors' goal is an HbA_{1C} of less than or equal to 8% prior to surgical reconstruction. In certain clinical settings, however, such as worsening of deformity with impending soft tissue compromise, instability, or acute neuropathic fracture dislocations, surgical reconstruction may be performed even if the HbA_{1C} is greater than 8%. The decision to intervene despite an elevated HbA_{1C} is made on a case-by-case basis. Postoperative glycemic control has also been shown to influence postoperative complications. A retrospective study of diabetic inpatients admitted after foot and ankle surgery evaluated random serum glucose measurements.[10] Patient were divided into 2 groups: those with a random serum glucose that was less than or equal to 200 mg/dL during their postoperative admission and those who had a random serum glucose greater than 200 mg/dL at some point during their admission. A random glucose of greater than 200 mg/dL was associated with a significantly increased risk of surgical site infection compared with patients whose glucose did not rise above 200 mg/dL. Approximately 12% of patients who had a random glucose greater than 200 mg/dL developed a surgical site infection postoperatively compared with approximately 5% in the group of patients who did not have a random glucose level of greater than 200 mg/dL ($P = .03$).[10] Postoperatively, hospital medicine comanagement of inpatients can provide optimal perioperative care.

Vitamin D

Serum vitamin D levels (serum 25-hydroxyvitamin D) should be evaluated preoperatively. Patients with values of less than 30 should receive vitamin D replacement with 50,000 IU (International units) weekly for 12 weeks ideally prior to reconstruction to optimize bone healing. Moore and colleagues[11] performed a case-matched study comparing 29 patients who underwent successful fusion to 29 patients who experienced nonunion after attempted foot fusion. Patients with vitamin D deficiency or insufficiency were 8.1 times more likely to develop a nonunion.[11] Yoho and colleagues[12] demonstrated significantly lower vitamin D levels (serum 25-hydroxyvitamin D) in patients with diabetes, both with and without CN, when compared with a cohort of nondiabetic patients.[12] Metabolic activation of vitamin D (vitamin D_3) initially takes place by hydroxylation in the liver, converting it to 25-hydroxyvitamin D_3.[13] The second step in bioactivation then occurs in the kidney where 25-hydroxyvitamin D_3 is converted to 1α-dihydroxyvitamin D_3.[13] In patients with CN and concomitant renal disease, vitamin D deficiency is common. Complete blood cell count (CBC) should be obtained to evaluate for potential anemia.

Additional Lab Testing

Albumin and prealbumin are protein makers of nutritional status and can help determine if nutritional optimization is necessary perioperatively. When a wound is present and infection is a concern, erythrocyte sedimentation rate (ESR) and C-reactive protein (CRP) are inflammatory markers that can help detect presence of infection as well as patient response to antibiotic therapy.

Preoperative Imaging

Full weight-bearing radiographs of the foot and ankle allow visualization of the location and extent of the CN deformity. Hindfoot alignment views help fully assess the position of the calcaneus relative to the distal tibia. A previous study of 114 patients with mid-foot CN found that sagittal plane deformities were more likely to be associated with DFU in CN patients.[14] CN patients with DFU had significantly greater deformity when evaluating the lateral talar first metatarsal angle, calcaneal pitch, cuboid height, medial column height, calcaneal fifth metatarsal angle, talar declination, and lateral tibiotalar angle on weight-bearing radiographs.[14] Lateral column deformity was associated with worse outcomes, and this can be identified radiographically by a decrease in the cuboid height, decreased calcaneal pitch, and decreased lateral calcaneal fifth metatarsal angle.[14] Restoration of these radiographic parameters is an important part of intraoperative reconstruction and is discussed later in this review. MRI may be a helpful tool to identify all affected regions of the foot and ankle that may appear normal or without neuropathic changes on radiographs. Meacock and colleagues[15] proposed a bone marrow edema and fracture scoring system after studying a group of patients with acute CN who underwent MRI. Their method can be used to grade the extent of destruction in the active CN foot.[15] MRI may help the surgeon plan for fusion that extends past the zone of injury, potentially providing more stability.[16] CT may provide further 3-D detail for surgical planning.

Preoperative Patient Discussion

Once a patient has been medically optimized for surgical intervention, it is critical to ensure that the patient understands the goals of surgery and the postoperative recovery course. Defining realistic expectations is critical. Complications are frequent and despite successful surgical intervention (plantigrade foot, ulcer-free, able to wear shoes, and braceable) some patients may not be able to return to their pre-Charcot activity level. In some cases, complications associated with surgery may result in minor or major amputations. Preoperative and postoperative patient function can be evaluated with patient-reported outcome measurement instruments, such as the Foot and Ankle Ability Measure or Medical Outcomes Study Short Form 36.[17–19] A recent review revealed that there is no gold standard instrument to measure outcomes in this patient population[20]

Another useful preoperative tool is borrowed from surgeons specializing in adult reconstruction and sports medicine. Outpatient pre-surgery rehabilitation referral (ie, PREHAB) for physical therapy and occupational therapy is useful to improve proprioception, balance, and muscle strength and to identify what type of mobility aids may be necessary postoperatively. This also can facilitate discharge to home or identify patients who require skilled nursing placement after surgery. In an effort to safely reduce length of stay, judicious PREHAB may be an important component in the pre-operative planning period.

PART 2: SURGICAL INTERVENTION

The goal of surgery is to achieve a stable, well-aligned, plantigrade foot and ankle that permits ambulation. Anatomic osseous realignment should allow for even distribution of forces once a patient begins to ambulate, potentially preventing future recurrence of the CN deformity. Surgical reconstruction usually consists of a combination of tendon releases/lengthening, fusions, and osteotomies as needed to address the deformity. Sammarco[16] originally discussed the concept of "superconstructs" in CN surgical reconstruction, in order to improve stability and decrease the chances of failure.[16] Four principles define this concept. First, the fusion should extend past the zone of injury to include joints that are not involved. Second, enough bone should be resected to allow for reduction of the deformity without soft tissue compromise. Third, the strongest device that can be tolerated by the bone and tissue should be used for fixation. Finally, fixation should be applied in a position that maximizes biomechanical stability.[16]

Soft Tissue Release

Release of contracted soft tissue structures is a critical part of deformity correction. Longstanding deformity leads to tissue contracture, necessitating release to fully correct the osseous CN deformity. The Achilles tendon often is contracted and often requires lengthening in the setting of midfoot/hindfoot CN reconstruction in order to decrease forces on the midfoot region. This may be performed percutaneously or open via 3 small incisions, depending on surgeon preference. In the setting of a varus deformity, the posterior tibial tendon may require complete release or lengthening to achieve proper reduction of the foot and ankle. If contracture is still present after posterior tibial lengthening or release, further release of the medial soft tissue structures as well as the subtalar joint may be needed. In the setting of a longstanding valgus deformity, the peroneal tendons may require release or lengthening.

Osseous Correction: Midfoot

Intraoperative restoration of the talar–first metatarsal angle radiographically on both the anteroposterior (AP) and lateral views can be used to as a guide toward anatomic reduction during midfoot/hindfoot surgical reconstruction.[14] As discussed previously, calcaneal pitch, cuboid height, medial column height, calcaneal fifth metatarsal angle, talar declination, and lateral tibiotalar angles should be restored as close as possible to normal to fully correct any medial column and/or lateral column deformity.[14] A key study by Grant and colleagues[21] evaluated intramedullary beaming of the medial and lateral columns for diabetic CN reconstruction.[21] They concluded that intramedullary fixation/beaming both the medial and lateral columns allows for maximum control of the transverse arch of the foot and that additional fusion of the subtalar joint may also add further stabilization by limiting frontal and transverse plane torsion.[21] Creating a "superconstruct" that spans the zone of injury. It is important to note that realignment of the medial column may require subsequent "balancing" or realignment of the lateral column in order to place the foot in a plantigrade position. The authors typically remove the deformed medial bone as needed (eg, a subluxed navicular or deformed cuneiforms) to restore the AP and lateral talar–first metatarsal angle intraoperatively. An extensile medial incision will allow access to all medial joints and also the subtalar joint. In certain cases, the calcaneocuboid joint may be visualized through a medial incision. The excised bone segments, if viable, are placed on the back table and reimplanted as autograft as needed. If the bone that has been excised is no longer viable due to severe CN, an allograft may be used to reconstruct the defect (ie femoral head allograft). Once the medial column has been prepared for fusion, attention is directed to the lateral column where the joints are prepared as needed for fusion. Lateral column deformity or collapse must be addressed to restore lateral column alignment. To "balance" the medial column, the lateral column may require shortening. This may be accomplished by removal of osseous segments (such as a portion of the cuboid) as needed, to align with the medial column. Some surgeons achieve osseous correction by resecting multiplanar wedges of bone, rather than removal/realignment of bone. Once the medial and lateral columns have been prepared, temporary fixation can be used to maintain the reduction prior to definitive fixation. As the first step of reduction, the authors often place a Steinmann pin into the calcaneus as a "joystick", manually restoring the calcaneal inclination angle under fluoroscopic guidance. While maintaining the calcaneus in proper position using the joystick, another temporary

Steinman pin is then placed in a transarticular fashion from the plantar calcaneus, through the subtalar joint and across the tibiotalar joint. This ensures that the ankle and hindfoot are in the proper position during the remainder of the procedure. After this provisional fixation of the ankle and hindfoot, the authors proceed with fixation of the medial column by placing a guidewire for intramedullary fixation extending from the first metatarsal head into the talus. Additional intramedually fixation may be placed in the lesser metatarsals and into the hindfoot as needed. The authors have found that, ideally, 2 intramedullary (IM) screws that extend into the talus provide improved rotational stability. Another option to improve rotational stability is to use a plantar/medial neutralization plate in addition to the medial column intramedullary fixation. The prepared joints of the lateral column should be fixated as needed. Care should be taken to leave room in the talus for a subtalar screw if this joint has also been prepared for fusion. The authors generally fuse the subtalar joint in addition to the medial and lateral columns. As Grant and colleagues[21] have suggested, fusion of the medial column, lateral column, and subtalar joint may provide the most stability and potentially reduce the rate of recurrence and nonunion. A systematic review on midfoot CN surgical interventions show that there is much variability of in regards to surgical techniques and approaches.[22] In cases of concern for infection, external fixation is recommended.

Osseous Correction: Ankle/Hindfoot

Over the past few years, the most common anatomic locations for CN surgical intervention were the hindfoot (41.6%) and the ankle (38.4%), which may be because these regions are less amenable to bracing and conservative care.[23] A systematic review of 860 CN surgical cases identified 170 cases involving tibiotalocalcaneal (TTC) arthrodesis, which was approximately 20% of the surgeries performed for CN.[24] Surgeons should be experienced with various approaches to the ankle and hindfoot, because the soft tissue envelope quality determines which incisional approach may be used. As with midfoot reconstruction, choice of fixation is dependent on surgeon experience and soft tissue concerns (ulceration or infection). When there is no concern for infection, internal fixation may be used for TTC or pantalar arthrodesis. External fixation is used in settings where there is concern for infection, ulceration, or poor bone quality. In cases of talar insufficiency and collapse, with no ulceration or concern for infection, a femoral head allograft may be used to replace the talus[25] (**Figs. 2** and **3**).

Fixation Optimization: Internal Fixation

There are many options for internal fixation, including locking plates, screws, and intramedullary beaming/bolt options. Regardless of the method of fixation, the key is to provide enough fixation to maintain osseous alignment and achieve fusion. Intramedullary (IM) for CN midfoot reconstruction has increased in popularity. The intramedullary fixation works by sharing the load with the osseous and ligamentous structures of the foot, thereby helping the bone maintain anatomic alignment.[21] There has been a recent development in Charcot-specific fixation; however, there are no clinical studies reporting on the long-term surgical outcomes using these CN-specific devices over traditional methods of fixation. In general, the largest and strongest device that is tolerated by the bone and soft tissue should be selected. Retrograde IM hindfoot nail fixation for ankle and hindfoot CN correction increased in utilization. There are various retrograde IM hindfoot nail designs to select from, with some allowing for internal and or external fusion site compression as well as straight and slight valgus bend designs. Stress reaction or fracture of the

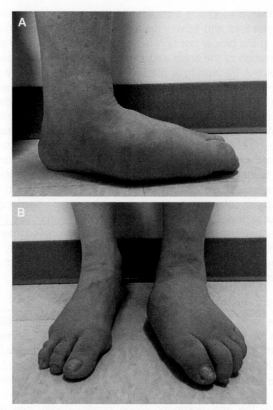

Fig. 2. (*A*, *B*) Preoperative clinical photos of patient with CN midfoot deformity.

tibia is a potential complication of retrograde IM nail fixation. The length of the IM nail is another important consideration. A previous cadaveric study on TTC arthrodesis reported on the biomechanics of IM nail length and stress reaction of the tibia.[26] They compared standard-length (150-mm) hindfoot IM nails to longer nails that ended in the proximal tibial metaphysis and found that a TTC fusion with a standard-length locked IM nail increased stress concentration at the proximal screw holes. This was not observed in the longer nails that terminated in the proximal tibial metaphysis, suggesting that a longer nail may help avoid tibial stress reaction/fracture in patients with osteopenia.[26] A study of 117 patients with an average follow-up of 2.5 years who underwent TTC arthrodesis with a retrograde IM nail found that 4 patients in the series with DM (3.4%) developed a fracture of the tibia at or above the proximal tip of the nail when a 150-mm nail was used.[25] Because of this potential complication, IM nails that engage the isthmus of the tibia can be used in high-risk patients. The surgeon must be comfortable with freehand insertion of the proximal interlocking screws when using a longer nail. In addition to the retrograde IM hindfoot nail, a supplemental screw may be placed across the ankle and/or subtalar joint. In the setting of talar collapse/destruction, femoral head allograft may be used to replace a deficient talus. Although the likelihood of limb salvage is high, the use of femoral head allograft has been shown to increase the risk of complication when used in patients undergoing TTC fusion.[25] In general,

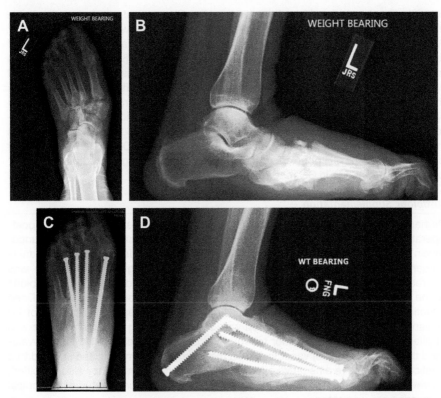

Fig. 3. (*A–D*) Preoperative and postoperative midfoot CN reconstruction: weight-bearing preoperative (*A, B*) and postoperative (*C, D*) radiographs demonstrating anatomic realignment and the authors' preferred internal fixation construct for midfoot CN reconstruction.

diabetic patients with CN who undergo TTC fusion with a retrograde IM nail have a good limb salvage rate.[25,27–30]

Fixation Optimization: External Fixation

External fixation often is used for reconstruction in the setting of ulceration or concern for infection. A series of 178 patients with CN underwent single-stage infection resection and CN deformity correction with the use of an external fixator.[31] Approximately 96% of patients achieved limb salvage.[31] Some investigators suggest the use of external fixation as supplemental fixation, in addition to internal fixation for CN reconstruction.[32] Although external fixation is an important method of fixation in Charcot patients, complications, such as pin tract infections can occur. In a retrospective review, patients with DM who underwent external fixator application experienced a 7-fold risk of wire complications compared with patients without DM.[23] Further studies are needed to determine if reconstruction using internal fixation supplemented with the addition of an external fixator increases healing rates in CN reconstruction.

Orthobiologic Supplementation

Although autogenous bone grafting is considered the gold advances have been made in orthobiologic development in recent years that may have a role in improvement of CN reconstruction fusion rates. A prospective study using bone marrow aspirate and platelet-rich plasma for 44 patients undergoing CN surgical correction showed a 91.3% fusion rate in this high-risk population; however, there was no control group.[33] A prospective, randomized, multicenter, controlled clinical trial evaluated the use of recombinant human platelet-derived growth factor-BB and β-tricalcium phosphate (rhPDGF-BB/β-TCP) for ankle and/or hindfoot arthrodesis. This group was compared with a group of patients undergoing arthrodesis with autograft. Patients treated with rhPDGF-BB/β-TCP had comparable hindfoot/ankle fusion rates to those treated with autograft.[34] A randomized study compared 75 patients undergoing ankle or hindfoot fusion using either rhPDGF-BB/β-TCP or autograft and found similar fusion rates in both groups.[35] To the best of the authors' knowledge, rhPDGF-BB/β-TCP has not been studied in the CN population. In the future, these bioengineered products may play an important role in CN reconstruction.

Antibiotic Supplementation

Perhaps one of the easiest and most cost-effective measures to help minimize postoperative infection development is the intraoperative application of topical vancomycin to the surgical site.[36] In a study of DM patients undergoing foot and ankle surgery, the overall likelihood of the development of surgical site infection was decreased by 73% in patients who received topically applied vancomycin antibiotic at the time of surgery, in addition to standard systemic antibiotic prophylaxis. Deep infection was 80% less likely in patients who received this treatment. The cost of 1 g of vancomycin at the study institution was $5.00, and 0.5 g to 1 g of powder was applied to the surgical sites prior to wound closure.[36] Chu and colleagues[37] evaluated the effects of topical vancomycin on mesenchymal stem cells and showed that application may have a negative effect on mesenchymal stems. They also specified, however, that this may be related to the amount applied. Further studies on topical antibiotics are warranted.[37]

Early Surgical Intervention

The ideal timing for surgical intervention is still not clear. Most surgical interventions take place during the nonacute phase, and this is based on historical concerns generated decades ago.[24] Surgical correction during the acute phase may allow for reconstruction before severe deformity develops, allowing for potentially "easier" anatomic realignment possibly leading to better long-term outcomes. Few studies have evaluated surgical correction in the acute phase,[38] and this may be a potential area of further research.

Postoperative Care

Postoperative visits should be frequent (ie, every 1–2 weeks) for close monitoring. CN reconstruction patients should remain non–weight bearing for longer than non-neuropathic patients. The authors typically keep patients immobilized (posterior splint, cast, total contact cast, and so forth) and non–weight bearing for at least 12 weeks post-operatively, until radiographic signs of fusion are evident. The use of a knee walker is especially helpful for patients. Once there are radiographic signs that bone healing is occurring, protected weight bearing can be started in a total contact cast with eventual transition to a removable walking boot. Once patients are ambulatory in a removable boot, and there are no signs of reconstruction failure, the authors typically have them evaluated for custom bracing. There are multiple bracing options, such as a Charcot restraint orthotic walker or double upright ankle-foot orthosis. In the authors experience, it is key to protect the patient in bracing for 1 year to 2 years postoperatively or even lifelong. Many patients benefit from physical therapy after the immobilization period has ended.

Health Care Economics

Caring for patients with diabetes-related foot complications, such as CN, is costly. Although there have been changes in the Affordable Care Act (ACA), the federal government and third-party payers will play an increasingly important role in reimbursement to providers and hospitals. Key provisions of the ACA are to improve quality, control the rising health care costs, and encourage wellness and prevention. Accountable care organizations have been established to achieve the goals of the ACA, and surgeons who treat CN will be expected to be responsible citizens in managing these complex patients. This is a period of transition from volume-based care to value-based care, and the mandate is to demonstrate high-quality outcomes while controlling costs. Patients are complex and often experience higher rates of complications and readmissions, and surgeons will be held accountable for these. Consequently, optimizing patient comorbidities and perioperative care will be critical to achieving these goals. Surgeons will need to demonstrate that what they do is high quality and cost effective and should encourage multicenter collaboration to study this relatively uncommon (but not rare) disease. It does not take much imagination to foresee the day when the health care system determines what type of fixation and bioengineered products can be used for a CN reconstruction. This already has occurred in adult reconstructive surgery (hip and knee replacement) and spine surgery (implants), where hospitals determine what type of implants can be used. Implant costs represent approximately 70% of hospital costs for major orthopedic procedures, and, consequently, cutting implant costs are one of the major ways to reduce overall costs. Other cost reduction measures include reducing the length of stay and reducing the rate of readmission.

SUMMARY

CN reconstruction is a challenge even for the most seasoned foot and ankle surgeon. Multiple studies have demonstrated the negative impact of CN on patient quality of life.[18,19] The ultimate goal should be to help improve patients' mental and physical well-being. Most recently, evaluation of patient-reported outcomes revealed that successful CN surgical reconstruction improved patient quality of life.[39] Patient selection, preoperative medical optimization, and a well-planned surgical intervention are key to optimizing reconstruction results. Surgeons should strive to provide high-quality, cost-effective care by optimizing patient selection and perioperative care. Objective measures of patient outcomes will become increasingly important with the transition to value-based care.

REFERENCES

1. Wukich DK, Crim BE, Frykberg RG, et al. Neuropathy and poorly controlled diabetes increase the rate of surgical site infection after foot and ankle surgery. J Bone Joint Surg Am 2014;96(10):832–9.

2. Gregg EW, Sorlie P, Paulose-Ram R, et al. Prevalence of lower-extremity disease in the US adult population >=40 years of age with and without diabetes: 1999-2000 national health and nutrition examination survey. Diabetes Care 2004; 27(7):1591–7.

3. Wukich DK, Raspovic KM, Suder NC. Prevalence of peripheral arterial disease in patients with diabetic charcot neuroarthropathy. J Foot Ankle Surg 2016;55(4):727–31.

4. Wukich DK, Shen W, Raspovic KM, et al. Noninvasive arterial testing in patients with diabetes: a guide for foot and ankle surgeons. Foot Ankle Int 2015;36(12): 1391–9.

5. Williams DT, Harding KG, Price P. An evaluation of the efficacy of methods used in screening for lower-limb arterial disease in diabetes. Diabetes Care 2005;28(9): 2206–10.

6. Brooks B, Dean R, Patel S, et al. TBI or not TBI: that is the question. Is it better to measure toe pressure than ankle pressure in diabetic patients? Diabet Med 2001; 18(7):528–32.

7. Andersen CA. Noninvasive assessment of lower extremity hemodynamics in individuals with diabetes mellitus. J Vasc Surg 2010;52(3 Suppl):76S–80S.

8. Cao P, Eckstein HH, De Rango P, et al. Chapter II: diagnostic methods. Eur J Vasc Endovasc Surg 2011;42(Suppl 2):S13–32.

9. Norgren L, Hiatt WR, Dormandy JA, et al. Inter-society consensus for the management of peripheral arterial disease (TASC II). Eur J Vasc Endovasc Surg 2007;33(Suppl 1):S1–75.

10. Sadoskas D, Suder NC, Wukich DK. Perioperative glycemic control and the effect on surgical site infections in diabetic patients undergoing foot and ankle surgery. Foot Ankle Spec 2016;9(1):24–30.

11. Moore KR, Howell MA, Saltrick KR, et al. Risk factors associated with nonunion after elective foot and ankle reconstruction: a case-control study. J Foot Ankle Surg 2017;56(3):457–62.

12. Yoho RM, Frerichs J, Dodson NB, et al. A comparison of vitamin D levels in nondiabetic and diabetic patient populations. J Am Podiatr Med Assoc 2009;99(1): 35–41.

13. Dusso AS, Brown AJ, Slatopolsky E. Vitamin D. Am J Physiol Renal Physiol 2005; 289(1):F8–28.

14. Wukich DK, Raspovic KM, Hobizal KB, et al. Radiographic analysis of diabetic midfoot charcot neuroarthropathy with and without midfoot ulceration. Foot Ankle Int 2014;35(11):1108–15.

15. Meacock L, Petrova NL, Donaldson A, et al. Novel semiquantitative bone marrow oedema score and fracture score for the magnetic resonance imaging assessment of the active charcot foot in diabetes. J Diabetes Res 2017;2017:8504137.

16. Sammarco VJ. Superconstructs in the treatment of charcot foot deformity: plantar plating, locked plating, and axial screw fixation. Foot Ankle Clin 2009;14(3): 393–407.

17. Martin RL, Irrgang JJ, Burdett RG, et al. Evidence of validity for the foot and ankle ability measure (FAAM). Foot Ankle Int 2005;26(11):968–83.

18. Raspovic KM, Wukich DK. Self-reported quality of life in patients with diabetes: a comparison of patients with and without Charcot neuroarthropathy. Foot Ankle Int 2014;35(3):195–200.

19. Pinzur MS, Evans A. Health-related quality of life in patients with Charcot foot. Am J Orthop (Belle Mead NJ) 2003;32(10):492–6.

20. Hogg FR, Peach G, Price P, et al. Measures of health-related quality of life in diabetes-related foot disease: a systematic review. Diabetologia 2012;55(3): 552–65.

21. Grant WP, Garcia-Lavin S, Sabo R. Beaming the columns for Charcot diabetic foot reconstruction: a retrospective analysis. J Foot Ankle Surg 2011;50(2):182–9.

22. Shazadeh Safavi P, Jupiter DC, Panchbhavi V. A systematic review of current surgical interventions for charcot neuroarthropathy of the midfoot. J Foot Ankle Surg 2017;56(6):1249–52.

23. Wukich DK, Belczyk RJ, Burns PR, et al. Complications encountered with circular ring fixation in persons with diabetes mellitus. Foot Ankle Int 2008;29(10): 994–1000.

24. Schneekloth BJ, Lowery NJ, Wukich DK. Charcot neuroarthropathy in patients with diabetes: an updated systematic review of surgical management. J Foot Ankle Surg 2016;55(3):586–90.

25. Wukich DK, Mallory BR, Suder NC, et al. Tibiotalocalcaneal arthrodesis using retrograde intramedullary nail fixation: comparison of patients with and without diabetes mellitus. J Foot Ankle Surg 2015;54(5):876–82.

26. Noonan T, Pinzur M, Paxinos O, et al. Tibiotalocalcaneal arthrodesis with a retrograde intramedullary nail: a biomechanical analysis of the effect of nail length. Foot Ankle Int 2005;26(4):304–8.

27. Chraim M, Krenn S, Alrabai HM, et al. Mid-term follow-up of patients with hindfoot arthrodesis with retrograde compression intramedullary nail in Charcot neuroarthropathy of the hindfoot. Bone Joint J 2018;100-B(2):190–6.

28. Caravaggi CM, Sganzaroli AB, Galenda P, et al. Long-term follow-up of tibiocalcaneal arthrodesis in diabetic patients with early chronic Charcot osteoarthropathy. J Foot Ankle Surg 2012;51(4):408–11.

29. Pinzur MS, Kelikian A. Charcot ankle fusion with a retrograde locked intramedullary nail. Foot Ankle Int 1997;18(11):699–704.

30. Vasukutty N, Jawalkar H, Anugraha A, et al. Correction of ankle and hind foot deformity in Charcot neuroarthropathy using a retrograde hind foot nail-The Kings' Experience. Foot Ankle Surg 2018;24(5):406–10.

31. Pinzur MS, Gil J, Belmares J. Treatment of osteomyelitis in charcot foot with single-stage resection of infection, correction of deformity, and maintenance with ring fixation. Foot Ankle Int 2012;33(12):1069–74.

32. Hegewald KW, Wilder ML, Chappell TM, et al. Combined internal and external fixation for diabetic charcot reconstruction: a retrospective case series. J Foot Ankle Surg 2016;55(3):619–27.

33. Pinzur MS. Use of platelet-rich concentrate and bone marrow aspirate in high-risk patients with Charcot arthropathy of the foot. Foot Ankle Int 2009;30(2):124–7.

34. DiGiovanni CW, Lin SS, Baumhauer JF, et al. Recombinant human platelet-derived growth factor-BB and beta-tricalcium phosphate (rhPDGF-BB/beta-TCP): an alternative to autogenous bone graft. J Bone Joint Surg Am 2013; 95(13):1184–92.

35. Daniels TR, Younger AS, Penner MJ, et al. Prospective randomized controlled trial of hindfoot and ankle fusions treated with rhPDGF-BB in combination with a beta-TCP-collagen matrix. Foot Ankle Int 2015;36(7):739–48.

36. Wukich DK, Dikis JW, Monaco SJ, et al. Topically applied vancomycin powder reduces the rate of surgical site infection in diabetic patients undergoing foot and ankle surgery. Foot Ankle Int 2015;36(9):1017–24.

37. Chu S, Chen N, Dang ABC, et al. The effects of topical vancomycin on mesenchymal stem cells: more may not Be better. Int J Spine Surg 2017;11:12.

38. Simon SR, Tejwani SG, Wilson DL, et al. Arthrodesis as an early alternative to nonoperative management of charcot arthropathy of the diabetic foot. J Bone Joint Surg Am 2000;82-A(7):939–50.

39. Kroin E, Chaharbakhshi EO, Schiff A, et al. Improvement in quality of life following operative correction of midtarsal charcot foot deformity. Foot Ankle Int 2018; 39(7):808–11.

Lower Extremity Amputations in At-Risk Patients

A Focus on Tissue Viability and Function in the Compromised Limb

Vikas S. Kotha, BS[a], Kevin Ragothaman, DPM[a,b],
Elliot Walters, MD[a], Christopher E. Attinger, MD[a],
John S. Steinberg, DPM[a,*]

KEYWORDS

- Amputation • Limb salvage • Team approach • Functional surgery

KEY POINTS

- Pedal amputations are commonly performed in the diabetic population.
- A team approach is paramount to ensure multifaceted care for the complex patient at risk for limb loss.
- Amputations require careful surgical planning, attention to functional biomechanics, and close follow-up to minimize reulceration and reamputation.
- Evaluation of patient quality of life and functional ability is an important part of the surgical planning process.

INTRODUCTION

Limb loss is an issue that plagues our health care system, debilitating both patients and the health care industry. An estimated 185,000 amputations occur in the United States every year, with vascular disease being the predominant reason for amputations in individuals 65 years and older.[1,2] Although there are instances when a patient may benefit from a well-performed below-the-knee amputation, such as younger and more active patients or those who have sustained extensive tissue loss, a recent study revealed that patient's fear loss of a limb greater than death.[3]

Disclosure Statement: None of the authors have relevant conflict of interest to disclose.
[a] Department of Plastic and Reconstructive Surgery, Center for Wound Healing, MedStar Georgetown University Hospital, 3800 Reservoir Road Northwest, Washington, DC 20007, USA;
[b] Division of Podiatric Surgery, MedStar Washington Hospital Center, MedStar Georgetown University Hospital, 3800 Reservoir Road Northwest, Washington, DC 20007, USA
* Corresponding author.
E-mail address: John.Steinberg@medstar.net

Unfortunately, minor foot amputations are often met with disregard and are approached with improper preparation. It is crucial to recognize the complexity of these patients' condition and to approach any amputation procedure with care and great attention to detail to achieve the best long-term success possible. In a study of 126 patients who underwent such amputations, 43% were found to develop a postoperative infection.[4] Another study found the 30-day readmission rate in a cohort of 219 minor amputations to be 5%, with 37% of the cohort needing reoperation.[5]

To prevent postoperative complications, thorough surgical planning is warranted for all foot amputations. This includes examination of vascularity, infection status, and close attention to biomechanical deformity. All efforts for limb preservation must be met with consideration of quality of life and a follow-up plan for postoperative care. These patients must be educated early of their risk for limb loss as a complication from any amputation surgery.

A PATIENT-FOCUSED APPROACH TO PEDAL AMPUTATIONS

When minor amputations are pursued in patients who are at risk for limb loss, all efforts must be made with consideration of quality of life. Emergent infection in the setting of sepsis necessitates swift operative debridement and intravenous antibiotics to preserve life. In these cases, proximity of infection dictates level of amputation, and consideration should be paid to preserving as much tissue as possible. Removal of nonviable, necrotic tissue, and decompression of infected compartments, allowing for drainage of purulence, are paramount during this initial operative debridement (**Fig. 1**). Although a tourniquet may be applied and inflated in the case of excessive bleeding, we recommend minimal use to assess tissue viability and perfusion intraoperatively (see **Fig. 1**).

Following decompression and debridement of infected, devitalized tissue, and preservation of healthy tissue, a biomechanical evaluation is imperative to maintain a functional limb. Understanding patient goals and expectations gives the provider insight into amputation-level decisions and the risk-to-benefit ratio of pursuing reconstructive surgery. Before wound closure, the patient's remaining tissue should be examined to ensure that they are left with a functional limb that minimizes reulceration and can tolerate weight-bearing (**Fig. 2**).

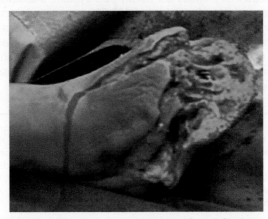

Fig. 1. Patient presenting with sepsis and necrotizing foot infection, which necessitated emergent surgery with exploration of affected compartments. In this instance, care should be taken to preserve as much healthy tissue as possible.

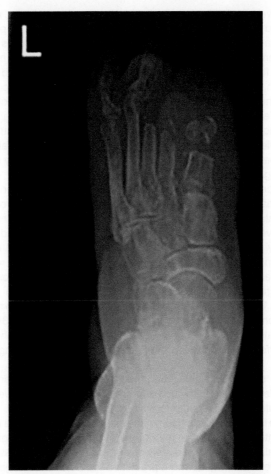

Fig. 2. After infection is eradicated, important consideration must be given to the functional viability of the foot. Preserving minor digits, sesamoids after partial ray resection, and disregarding the metatarsal parabola increase the risk of reulceration and reoperation.

PROGNOSTIC FACTORS TO DETERMINE AMPUTATION LEVEL

Several attempts have been made to develop classification systems and determine prognostic markers that will predict amputation risk in patients with diabetic foot ulcers. As has often been described, diabetic foot ulcers tend to be multifactorial.[6] In addition, the presence or absence of other comorbidities (ie, peripheral arterial disease or end-stage renal disease) may drastically alter the prognosis.[7]

The most widely known system is the Society for Vascular Surgery Wound, Ischemia, and foot Infection (WIfI) classification system. Introduced in 2013, this system was designed by expert consensus on the major factors leading to amputation in threatened limbs, especially in diabetics.[8–10] Patient amputation risk at 1 year is stratified based on individual scores for wound depth and location, ischemic grade (based on noninvasive methods), and infection grade. The composite of these 3 scores places a patient into 1 of 4 clinical stages based on likelihood of amputation at 1 year: clinical stage 1, very low; clinical stage 2, low; clinical stage 3, moderate; clinical stage 4, high.[10,11]

Although relatively new, this classification system has been studied extensively both prospectively and retrospectively. Zhan and colleagues,[11] in 2015, published one of the earliest evaluations of the WIfI system. They reviewed the records of 257 patients, 83% of whom were diabetic, with 280 at-risk limbs in a prospectively maintained database. This study found a positive correlation between WIfI stage and both major and minor amputation. Weaver and colleagues[12] and Mathioudakis and colleagues[9] independently published more recent reviews of the WIfI system with exclusively patients with diabetes. Weaver found a positive correlation between WIfI staging and wound healing, but did not evaluate correlation between WIfI stage and amputation. Mathioudakis also identified positive correlation between WIfI stage and healing, but did not find correlation between stage and major amputation; however, they did find correlation between stage and risk of minor amputation.

This disparity between WIfI stage and major amputation prediction may be related to the reversible nature of ischemic grade as noted by Leithead and colleagues[10] in his retrospective evaluation of 172 critical limb ischemia patients receiving revascularization. Postoperative WIfI restaging was performed retrospectively and compared with the prospectively performed preoperative WIfI staging. They found on preoperative staging only wound grade correlated significantly with amputation ($P = .03$). However, 1-month postoperative restaging correlated strongly to amputation for advanced wound grade (grade >1, odds ratio [OR] = 10.18, $P<.001$) and infection grade (grade >0, OR = 17.86, $P<.001$). Ischemia grade is not correlated to amputation until restaging at 6 months postintervention (grade >1, OR = 5.74, $P = .039$). This likely reflects the high rate of vascular reintervention performed in this cohort (30.1%). No analysis was performed for nonvascular interventions or considering the composite WIfI stage.

The Leithead study highlights the importance of postintervention restaging. Whereas both Weaver and Mathioudakis found no correlation between WIfI staging and major amputation, their patients were staged preintervention. Leithead noted that preoperative ischemia grade had no correlation to postoperative ischemia grade. They further pointed out that over the course of treatment WIfI staging improved at every time interval, including immediately postoperatively. This suggests that the trend of WIfI stages over time may be more predictive than the initial stage itself.

Other systems have been proposed to predict amputation in patients with diabetic foot ulcers. A systematic review and meta-analysis of these systems was performed by Monteiro-Soares and colleagues[13] in 2013. This study evaluated 8 different classification systems for major and minor lower extremity amputation risk. Whereas some of these systems had prospective cohorts, none of the classification systems examined had robust data supporting their results. A 2016 systematic review by Brownrigg and colleagues[14] evaluated various prognostic markers for amputation. This review identified 11 studies with 5890 combined patients. Of the 8 different parameters they evaluated (ankle brachial index [ABI], ankle pressures, toe pressures, fluorescein toe slope, Doppler waveform analysis, TcPO$_2$, skin perfusion pressure, and pulse palpation), only the combination of ABI less than 0.5 and ankle pressure less than 50 mm Hg was predictive of amputation (relative risk = 25.0, 95% CI: 13.5–41.9). However, in the diabetic population this is not clinically useful because ABI has been shown to be unreliable.[15]

Thus far, the Society for Vascular Surgery WIfI classification system has the strongest evidence for early prediction of amputation but most studies examine heterogenous populations including diabetic and nonpatients with diabetes. Furthermore, few of these studies include analysis of the cause of the wound. Those studies that did restrict their wound population to diabetic foot ulcers failed to correlate WIfI stage to major amputation risk; further investigation is warranted. Regular reassessment after intervention is likely to strengthen the predictive value of the WIfI system. Other systems or individual measures have, thus far, failed to accurately predict 1-year progression to amputation or amputation-free survival. Because the patient with diabetes is a complex host with myriad complications and comorbidities, predicting those that will progress to amputation requires a multifaceted approach.

PERIOPERATIVE CONSIDERATIONS

Complex infection cases that require staged procedures before closure should be performed through a team approach. The surgical team may find input from infectious disease, internal medicine, physical and occupational therapists, prosthetists, and other medical and mental health specialties to be beneficial. After eradication of emergent infection, the opinion of these teams should be sought to plan hospital course and appropriate discharge.

Following the index operation, wounds can be dressed with negative pressure wound therapy (NPWT) dressing with instillation, which has been shown to decrease hospital length of stay and time to final closure compared with NPWT at standard settings.[16] When there is concern for postoperative bleeding or the anatomic site is not conducive to NPWT, the wound can be dressed with 1% acetic acid-soaked gauze that should be changed 2 to 3 times daily. Retention sutures can be used across raised flaps to prevent retraction of tissue from postoperative edema.

Predebridement and postdebridement deep tissue and bone cultures should be collected intraoperatively. The postdebridement cultures are followed in the postoperative period and guide antibiotic therapy as well as surgical planning. Controversy exists with regard to diagnosis of osteomyelitis by pathology and culture.[17] It is advisable to review culture and pathology results with relation to the clinical intraoperative assessment of bone condition.

Arterial perfusion should also be assessed in the interim. Although several noninvasive vascular testing methods exist, including ABI, duplex ultrasound, and transcutaneous oxygen pressure monitoring, an arteriogram is often indicated to best evaluate inflow to the wound and to treat macrovascular disease in a method targeting the angiosome of interest.[18] This information guides surgical decision-making with regard to handling of tissue, identifying high-risk patients, assessing risk-to-benefit ratio of reconstructive surgery, likelihood of wound healing, and level of amputation.

DIGITAL AND RAY AMPUTATION

Digital amputations are commonly performed in the diabetic population, with the most common cause being gangrene.[19] Toe amputations generally have good short-term outcomes, with 95% healing rate reported following toe amputations undergoing primary closure.[20] However, a prospective study of 245 patients undergoing digital amputation showed a 47.1% reamputation rate within 5 years, with HbA1c >9% and age older than 70 years identified as independent risk factors.[21] Phalangeal osteomyelitis is another common reason for toe amputation. In the setting of distal hallux infection, patients should be evaluated for hallux rigidus by physical examination and radiographically as it has been shown to increase likelihood of reamputation and may dictate a complete toe amputation instead of a partial toe amputation.[22]

Ray resection may be necessary for infection or gangrene present proximal to the metatarsophalangeal joints (MTPJs). Amputation of the first MTPJ leads to instability in the forward propulsion phase of gait, affecting walking speed and ankle, knee, and hip range of motion.[23] Plantar peak pressure is distributed beneath the neighboring metatarsal heads causing transfer lesions and potentially subsequent osteomyelitis of other rays of the foot. This is supported by a study that reported that 69% of patients who underwent partial first ray amputation developed a foot ulceration within a mean of 10.5 months, and 42.4% underwent more proximal amputation.[24] Proper custom shoes and accommodation is necessary when the patient begins weight-bearing following partial first ray amputation to help prevent complications.

Furthermore, sacrificing the attachment of the long flexor and extensor tendons to the hallux leads to destabilization at the knot of Henry and abnormal pull of the flexor digitorum longus tendons. This causes eventual contracture of the lesser digits and risks further ulceration. Prophylactic percutaneous flexor tendon release has shown positive results for preventing and treating toe ulcers and can be beneficial in this patient population.[25] If the halluceal flexor and extensor tendons are deemed viable with sufficient length, tenodesis can be performed in an attempt to prevent lesser digital contracture (**Fig. 3**).

Central ray amputations should be approached with consideration to the native parabola. The proximal base of the 2nd metatarsal and its articulations should be preserved in order to maintain the keystone stability of the midtarsal apparatus. Closure of the central ray is carried out after a clean-margin of bone yields negative results for osteomyelitis. A toe spacer can be inserted between remaining digits to prevent abductovalgus deformity to the first MTPJ following partial second ray amputation.

Lateral ray amputations become challenging when compromise of the fifth metatarsal styloid process occurs. Infection of the peroneus brevis and its insertion necessitates removal to prevent necrotizing infection along the lateral compartment of the lower extremity. Loss of peroneus brevis function and overpowering of the posterior tibial tendon and gastrocnemius-soleus complex causes adductovarus contracture. Boffeli and colleagues[26] have described a technique using transfer of the peroneus longus to the cuboid with a biotenodesis screw in a 2-staged approach using antibiotic-loaded polymethylmethacrylate beads in the interim. Fusion of the ankle joint may be necessary when rigid adductovarus contracture develops (**Fig. 4**).

TRANSMETATARSAL AMPUTATION

Tissue loss from infection or ischemia present proximal to the metatarsophalangeal joints often necessitates amputation at the level of the midfoot. Transmetatarsal

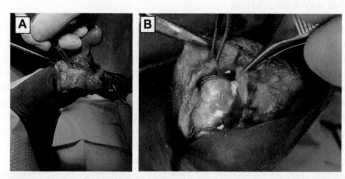

Fig. 3. First MTPJ disarticulation hallux amputation in individual with hallux gangrene and osteomyelitis of the distal phalanx (*A*). Identification of the halluceal flexor and extensor tendons for tenodesis to prevent contracture of the lesser digits (*B*). (*Courtesy of* Jacob Wynes, DPM, MS, Baltimore, MD.)

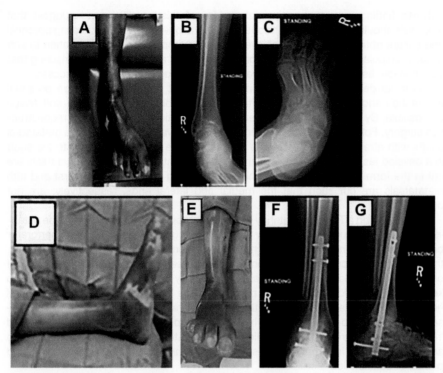

Fig. 4. (*A–D*) Rigid adductovarus contracture following complete fifth ray resection and free flap reconstruction. (*E–G*) Tibiotalocalcaneal arthrodesis was pursued through the transfibular approach with intramedullary fixation, Achilles tenectomy, and posteriomedial release, leading to painless ambulatory function with custom ankle-foot orthosis by 6 months postoperatively. (*Courtesy of* Caitlin S. Zarick, DPM, FACFAS, Washington D.C)

amputation (TMA) is a versatile procedure that provides the benefit of maintaining a metatarsal parabola to preserve native gait biomechanics. Because of the unstable nature of partial ray amputations noted earlier, it may be beneficial to consider TMA in ambulatory individuals when they have compromise distally of the first ray or multiple rays. Performing a TMA in this scenario can be more ideal for a well-perfused and bulky plantar flap to allow for weight-bearing with appropriate accommodation.

The functional benefits of TMA have been elucidated in previous studies. In a cohort of 394 comorbid patients with diabetes, 88% of whom were independent ambulators preoperatively, 77% were able to maintain their previous functional status at 12 months follow-up.[27] When assessed with the Locomotor Capability Index-5, Norvell and colleagues[28] found no significant decline in mobility in patients who underwent index TMA secondary to diabetes or vascular disease (n = 26). A 2001 study by Thomas and colleagues[29] reported that, although nearly 95% of patients with healed TMAs were able to independently ambulate by 7 months postoperatively, more than half of all index TMAs failed to heal and required reamputation.

Historically, the rate of healing following TMA has been reported to be low. In their 2011 study, Landry and colleagues[30] reported 53% of TMAs had successfully healed. In a study of 41 TMAs that failed to heal, all required proximal conversion within 3 months of index amputation 53.7% were converted to Chopart amputations, 24.4% to Lisfranc amputations, and 22% to major amputations.[31]

These findings reveal the complex nature of this condition and suggest that emphasis should be placed on intraoperative techniques to maximize healing potential and ensure optimal function is achieved following amputation. Strict attention to soft tissue manipulation, with consideration for viability of angiosomes, and ensuring that questionable tissue is removed before closure are crucial to achieving success.

The initial debridement of infection in a foot that is going to undergo potential amputation should be performed with the goal of preserving as much soft tissue as possible. By preserving length, there are more options in subsequent reconstructive surgery. Following full-thickness incision and elevation of flaps off the metatarsal shafts with atraumatic technique, the metatarsals are cut perpendicular to the shaft in a beveled fashion such that the plantar side is slightly shorter. The metatarsals are cut in the form of a parabola, with the second being the longest. The first and fifth metatarsals are cut such that the medial and lateral ends, respectively, are not prominent.

When planning a TMA, the patency of dorsal and plantar arterial flow must be established. The main source of blood flow for this procedure is the terminal deep perforator branch from the dorsalis pedis, which dives between the first and second metatarsal, thereby forming a critical arterial connection between the dorsal and plantar foot. If only the dorsalis pedis or the lateral plantar artery are patent, then it is critical to keep this connection intact. After performing the bone cuts, the first metatarsal head is removed medially such that the tissue between the first and second metatarsals is not visualized. The metatarsal heads are grasped with a towel clamp and turned 180° vertically toward the surgeon, allowing atraumatic dissection from the plantar flap and preserving the intermetatarsal tissue where connections between the dorsal and plantar circulation lie.

The second tarsometatarsal joint articulations are crucial for maintaining preservation of stability to the midfoot. The plantar plate apparatus should be removed with care to prevent damage of the underlying plantar metatarsal vessels. The sesamoids are removed as well. The ends of metatarsal shafts can be treated with electrocautery if they are bleeding or a patient is deemed to be at risk for developing heterotopic bone. Once debridement of all nonviable tissue is complete, we prefer to change gloves, drapes, and instruments before closure preparation to prevent contamination of the clean wound base.

A TMA needs to be well-balanced from a musculoskeletal standpoint to prevent reulceration on weight-bearing. As the insertions of the long extensor tendons are sacrificed, the posterior muscle group overpowers that of the ankle dorsiflexors, thus exacerbating tightness of the Achilles tendon. An equinovarus deformity develops because the tibialis anterior and posterior tibial tendon overpower the peroneus brevis. Failure to address musculoskeletal imbalance when performing a TMA, or in the postoperative period, increases the risk of failure. If the 4th and 5th flexor and extensor tendons are viable and adequate in length, the flexor can be tenodesed to its complementary extensor tendon with an absorbable monofilament suture to prevent varus deformity (**Fig. 5**). A percutaneous Achilles tendon lengthening can also be performed to weaken the plantar flexion forces across the ankle joint.

The plantar flap is frequently larger in diameter than the dorsal flap, which forms dog ears when closed. A wedge can be taken out from the central plantar flap so that the circumferences of both flaps are equal and symmetric closure is attained. We do not typically use absorbable suture to close deep tissue, but rather use monofilament nonabsorbable suture in vertical mattress fashion across the incision. When encountering a cross-T in a flap, an apical suture is used to prevent penetration of the apex of the flap with the needle (see **Fig. 5**).

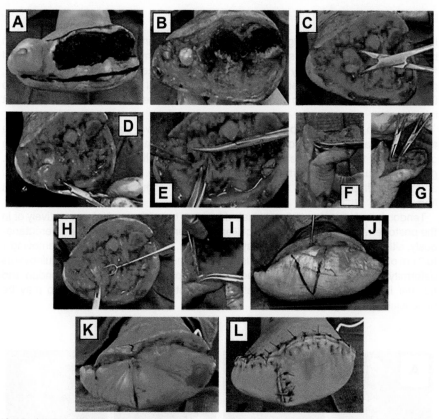

Fig. 5. (A) Debrided foot brought back to the operating room for transmetatarsal amputation. The open area has been painted with methylene blue to ensure that the debridement is adequate. (B, C) The fourth and fifth toes have been disarticulated and the reulceration of the rest of the foot has been excisionally debrided. The metatarsals must be recut to form a parabola with the second metatarsal being the longest. (D, E) The cut fifth metatarsal head is now being freed up from the surrounding tissue using a towel clamp. It is vertically flipped 180°, so that it can be dissected off the plantar soft tissue without destroying the underlying blood supply. (E, F) The volar plate is exposed by going into the flexor sheath with a tonsil or scissor. It is then cut along its center and both halves are removed taking care to stay on the plantar side to avoid the digital arteries. (G–I) To restore the dorsiflexion of the foot lost when the toes were amputated, one can tenodese the flexor and extensor of the fourth and/or fifth toes. Here, the flexors and extensor tendons of the fifth toe are located and placed on gentle traction (G). They are twisted together with the foot in neutral (H). They are then sewn together (H). (J–L) The plantar flap usually has a longer diameter than the dorsal flap. This inequality leads to dog ears on both sides. One can circumvent that by taking a large wedge from the center of the plantar flap to equalize the dorsal and plantar flap diameters. This then allows for simple closure with no dog ears.

A drain can be used in the setting of tissue dead space. We typically use an incisional NPWT dressing for up to 7 days postoperatively if there is adequate bleeding intraoperatively to minimize tension across the incision. We place the patient with the ankle in a neutral position in a well-padded posterior splint and keep them nonweight-bearing for at least 3 weeks. If the Achilles tendon is lengthened, we implement a walking boot when they are ambulatory for a total of 6 weeks from the date of surgery to prevent rupture (see **Fig. 5**).

LISFRANC AMPUTATION

If infection is proximal enough, one may find it necessary to perform an amputation by disarticulation at the tarsometatarsal joints. The same considerations for blood flow as described previously should be used to maximize success of this procedure, particularly with regard to removal of the first metatarsal medially and the second to fifth metatarsals laterally to prevent disturbing the deep plantar artery in the 1st interspace.

Once again, a proximal to distal approach with a towel clamp is used to remove the metatarsals. The keystone structure at the proximal second metatarsal base can be cut at the level of the cuneiforms to ensure stability at this junction; however, great care must be taken with the intermetatarsal tissue. When evaluating the dorsal and plantar flaps, the one with better vascularity should be preserved in length (**Fig. 6**).

Tendon imbalance should be evaluated and can be addressed intraoperatively or in the postoperative period. A tendo-Achilles lengthening can be performed percutaneously, although a frank tenectomy may be required, which is performed by removing 1 to 2 cm of the distal Achilles tendon just above its insertion to prevent late equinovarus deformity (**Fig. 7**). It may also be necessary to split the tibialis anterior tendon and transfer it to the cuboid. Alternatively, tibialis anterior tendon lengthening may be beneficial[32] (see **Fig. 7**).

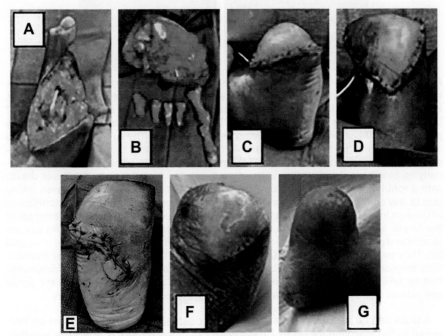

Fig. 6. (*A, B*) This patient presented with necrotizing fasciitis of the lateral forefoot. The soft tissue defect was quite large. We managed to preserve the hallux. At the follow-up operation to close the wound, we filleted the large toe. (*C, D*) The metatarsals were disarticulated at Lisfranc joint. The filleted flap was then rotated laterally to close the large defect. (*E–G*) The wound was closed and 2 cm of the distal Achilles tendon was resected. The amputation after 3 months.

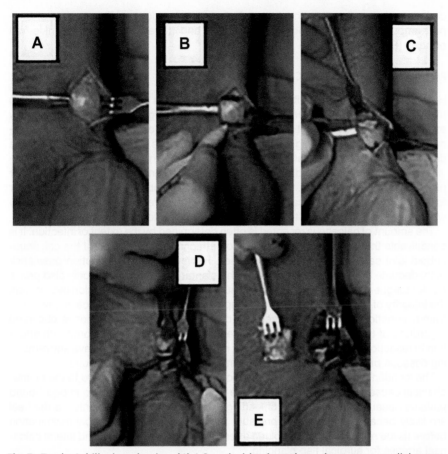

Fig. 7. Tendo-Achilles lengthening. (*A*) A 3-cm incision is made on the postero-medial aspect of the Achilles tendon 2 cm proximal to the Achilles insertion on the calcaneus. (*B*) The Achilles tendon is elevated above the plane of the skin and a 2-cm section is marked. (*C–E*) The tendon is transected sharply using either scalpel or scissors. The skin is closed primarily over the Achilles tendon defect.

CHOPART AMPUTATION

Amputation at the level of the midtarsal or Chopart joint is a difficult procedure to achieve favorable and functional results postoperatively, and is often used as a last effort before below-the-knee amputation. It is not a procedure to achieve function in athletic patients but can be useful in patients who are reliant on a limb to carry out activities of daily living, particularly if they already have an amputation on their contralateral limb.

Again, the blood flow must be assessed and the flap with better perfusion should be preserved in length. The flaps should be elevated in full-thickness fashion by staying directly on bone. It is easiest to perform the dorsal dissection and then peel each bone with a towel clamp to protect the plantar soft tissue. It is preferable to preserve as much plantar tissue as possible to cover the calcaneus and anterior talus. One must often be creative to use the best possible tissue to close this amputation.

An Achilles tenectomy must be performed concomitantly, with a small incision and resection of a 1- to 2-cm portion of the tendon. Ankle fusion may also be indicated for contracture recalcitrant to other tendon balancing procedures.[33] The success of Chopart amputation relies on postoperative care and a well-fitting custom ankle-foot orthosis (**Fig. 8**).

PARTIAL RESECTION OF CALCANEUS

Heel ulceration with concomitant calcaneal osteomyelitis are problematic and pose a high risk of major amputation.[34] Difficulty with offloading and impaired functionality exacerbate this issue. Partial calcanectomy has been shown to be an effective treatment as a method of avoiding major amputation, because resection of a portion of the calcaneus allows for removal of infected bone and wound closure. A systematic review of 16 publications found that 85% of reported patients are able to maintain their previous ambulatory status, and 83% are able to ambulate in custom shoegear following partial or total calcanectomy, although those receiving total calcanectomy were more likely to proceed to below-the-knee amputation.[35]

The amount of calcaneus resected is often determined by the extent of infection. It is conceivable that removal of Achilles tendon attachment or violation of the calcaneocuboid joint can destabilize foot mechanics. However, minimal resection poses risk of inadequate debridement. Removal of the plantar calcaneal cortex only also poses risk for tongue-type fracture of the calcaneus because the Achilles tendon overpowers the integrity of the dorsal cortex. Our group has found that no difference in Lower Extremity Function Score or increased risk of below-the-knee amputation is observed regardless of how much calcaneus is resected.[36] A partial calcanectomy with attention to resection of the vertical and plantar margins of the bone will relieve any remaining osseous prominence and facilitate primary closure of the heel wound.

The location of the wound can give adequate information with regard to the biomechanical causes. Wounds posterior to the heel are generally observed in bed-bound patients because of inadequate offloading, whereas those found plantar to the heel are likely because of increased pressure from calcaneal gait. Physical examination before tissue resection should include arterial Doppler of the medial and lateral calcaneal arteries for surgical flap planning.

The prone position is often necessary to properly perform the cardinal osteotomies with proper contouring. A Gaenslen-type incision is made to the level of bone to excise

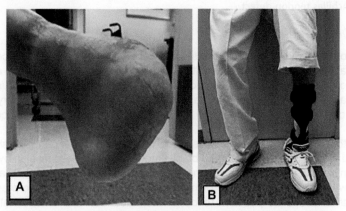

Fig. 8. Chopart amputation with Achilles tenectomy (A). Success of this amputation relies on appropriate bracing with custom ankle-foot orthosis and accommodative shoegear (B). (*Courtesy of* Tammer Elmarsafi, DPM, MBBCh, Washington D.C)

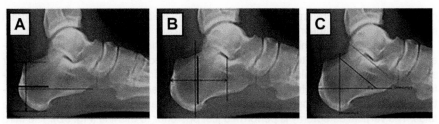

Fig. 9. Presurgical planning for the vertical contour calcanectomy. (*A*) A horizontal line (*thick line*) bisecting the superior and inferior aspect of the calcaneus posterior tuber is drawn. The horizontal arm of the calcaneal osteotomy is performed just inferior to this line. (*B*) A vertical line (*thick line*) bisecting the posterior aspect of the calcaneal tuber and the lateral talar process is drawn. The vertical arm of the calcaneal osteotomy is performed just posterior to this line. (*C*) An osteotomy is performed at 45° to the horizontal and vertical arms, parallel to the posterior facet of the subtalar joint.

the ulceration. The shape of the incision may vary based on the location of the heel ulcer. Full-thickness flaps are created to facilitate a well-perfused, durable closure. All nonviable soft tissue and bone are excised with wide margins and deep tissue and bone cultures are collected. If staged-closure is planned, an NPWT dressing

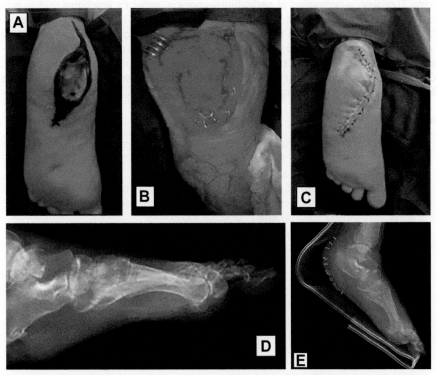

Fig. 10. (*A*) The wound is ellipsed in full-thickness fashion. (*B*) Medial and lateral flaps are raised. The posterior tuber of the calcaneus is resected, with special attention paid to contouring the poster and plantar margins. (*C*) The wound is closed with vertical mattress sutures with minimal tension. A drain may be inserted. (*D*) Preoperative imaging in patient with draining heel ulcer, with concern for acute osteomyelitis of the plantar posterior tuber of the calcaneus. (*E*) A heel-offloading splint is applied postoperatively.

may be applied with retention sutures to approximate the flaps and an arteriogram may be performed in the interim.

The 3 cardinal osteotomies are planned when reviewing lateral radiographs preoperatively. The first step is to draw the horizontal bisection of the superior and inferior aspect of the posterior calcaneal tuber (**Fig. 9**A). The first cardinal osteotomy is performed horizontally just inferior to this bisection. The second step is to draw the vertical bisection between the posterior calcaneal tuber and the lateral process of the talus. The vertical osteotomy is performed just posterior to this line (**Fig. 9**B). The third osteotomy is made parallel to the posterior facet of the subtalar joint (**Fig. 9**C). Following this, a power burr and hand rasp can be used to contour the posterior edge to allow for a smooth surface without osseous protuberance (**Fig. 10**).

Intraoperative fluoroscopy is useful to confirm adequate resection and structure of the calcaneus. A drain can be inserted because the cancellous bone from the calcaneus can lead to hematoma formation. An incisional NPWT dressing may be applied as well. The heel must be offloaded postoperatively with either a heel-offloading splint or external fixator device (see **Figs. 9** and **10**).

SUMMARY

Amputations distal to the ankle joint are commonly performed in efforts to preserve a limb. Thorough examination of pedal biomechanics, patient's functional status, and patient goals must be used to help prevent reulceration and further amputation. Once infection is resolved in the acute setting, musculotendon balancing should be used to maintain functionality of the limb. Patients should be closely followed postoperatively and monitored for biomechanical deformity that needs to be addressed. Careful attention to detail and adherence to surgical principles can help keep patients active and prevent further amputation.

REFERENCES

1. Ziegler-Graham K, MacKenzie E, Ephraim P, et al. Estimating the prevalence of limb loss in the United States: 2005 to 2050. Arch Phys Med Rehabil 2008. https://doi.org/10.1016/j.apmr.2007.11.005.
2. Dillingham TR, Pezzin LE, Mackenzie EJ. Limb amputation and limb deficiency: epidemiology and recent trends in the United States. South Med J 2002. https://doi.org/10.1097/00007611-200208000-00018.
3. Wukich DK, Raspovic KM, Suder NC. Patients with diabetic foot disease fear major lower-extremity amputation more than death. Foot Ankle Spec 2018. https://doi.org/10.1177/1938640017694722.
4. Uzzaman MM, Jukaku S, Kambal A, et al. Assessing the long-term outcomes of minor lower limb amputations: a 5-year study. Angiology 2011. https://doi.org/10.1177/0003319710395558.
5. Ries Z, Rungprai C, Harpole B, et al. Incidence, risk factors, and causes for thirty-day unplanned readmissions following primary lower-extremity amputation in patients with diabetes. J Bone Joint Surg Am 2014. https://doi.org/10.2106/JBJS.O.00449.
6. Jagadish M, McNally MM, Heidel RE, et al. Diabetic foot ulcers: the importance of patient comorbidity recognition and total contact casting in successful wound care. Am Surg 2016;82(8):733–6.
7. Ramanujam CL, Han D, Fowler S, et al. Impact of diabetes and comorbidities on split-thickness skin grafts for foot wounds. J Am Podiatr Med Assoc 2013. https://doi.org/10.7547/1030223.

8. Mills JL. Update and validation of the Society for Vascular Surgery Wound, Ischemia, and foot Infection threatened limb classification system. Semin Vasc Surg 2014. https://doi.org/10.1053/j.semvascsurg.2014.12.002.

9. Mathioudakis N, Hicks CW, Canner JK, et al. The Society for Vascular Surgery Wound, Ischemia, and foot Infection (WIfI) Classification System predicts wound healing but not major amputation in patients with diabetic foot ulcers treated in a multidisciplinary setting. J Vasc Surg 2017;65(6):1698–705.e1. https://doi.org/10.1016/j.jvs.2016.12.123.

10. Leithead C, Novak Z, Spangler E, et al. Importance of postprocedural Wound, Ischemia, and foot Infection (WIfI) restaging in predicting limb salvage. J Vasc Surg 2018. https://doi.org/10.1016/j.jvs.2017.07.109.

11. Zhan LX, Branco BC, Armstrong DG, et al. The Society for Vascular Surgery Lower Extremity Threatened Limb Classification System based on wound, ischemia, and foot infection (WIfI) correlates with risk of major amputation and time to wound healing. J Vasc Surg 2015. https://doi.org/10.1016/j.jvs.2014.11.045.

12. Weaver ML, Hicks CW, Canner JK, et al. The Society for Vascular Surgery Wound, Ischemia, and foot Infection (WIfI) Classification System predicts wound healing better than direct angiosome perfusion in diabetic foot wounds. J Vasc Surg 2018;68(5):1473–81.

13. Monteiro-Soares M, Boyko EJ, Ribeiro J, et al. Predictive factors for diabetic foot ulceration: a systematic review. Diabetes Metab Res Rev 2012;28(7):574–600.

14. Brownrigg JRW, Hinchliffe RJ, Apelqvist J, et al. Performance of prognostic markers in the prediction of wound healing or amputation among patients with foot ulcers in diabetes: a systematic review. Diabetes Metab Res Rev 2016. https://doi.org/10.1002/dmrr.2704.

15. Tehan PE, Bray A, Chuter VH. Non-invasive vascular assessment in the foot with diabetes: sensitivity and specificity of the ankle brachial index, toe brachial index and continuous wave Doppler for detecting peripheral arterial disease. J Diabetes Complications 2016. https://doi.org/10.1016/j.jdiacomp.2015.07.019.

16. Kim PJ, Attinger CE, Steinberg JS, et al. The impact of negative-pressure wound therapy with instillation compared with standard negative-pressure wound therapy: a retrospective, historical, cohort, controlled study. Plast Reconstr Surg 2014. https://doi.org/10.1097/01.prs.0000438060.46290.7a.

17. Meyr AJ, Singh S, Zhang X, et al. Statistical reliability of bone biopsy for the diagnosis of diabetic foot osteomyelitis. J Foot Ankle Surg 2011. https://doi.org/10.1053/j.jfas.2011.08.005.

18. Moulik PK, Mtonga R, Gill GV. Amputation and mortality in new-onset diabetic foot ulcers stratified by etiology. Diabetes Care 2003;26(2):491–4.

19. Jain AK, Varma A, Kumar H, et al. Digital amputations in the diabetic foot. J Diabet Foot Complications 2010;2(1):12–7.

20. Lakstein D, Lipkin A, Schorr L, et al. Primary closure of elective toe amputations in the diabetic foot—is it safe? J Am Podiatr Med Assoc 2014. https://doi.org/10.7547/0003-0538-104.4.383.

21. Chu YJ, Li XW, Wang PH, et al. Clinical outcomes of toe amputation in patients with type 2 diabetes in Tianjin, China. Int Wound J 2016. https://doi.org/10.1111/iwj.12249.

22. Oliver NG, Attinger CE, Steinberg JS, et al. Influence of hallux rigidus on reamputation in patients with diabetes mellitus after partial hallux amputation. J Foot Ankle Surg 2015. https://doi.org/10.1053/j.jfas.2015.06.007.

23. Aprile I, Galli M, Pitocco D, et al. Does first ray amputation in diabetic patients influence gait and quality of life? J Foot Ankle Surg 2018;57(1):44–51.
24. Borkosky SL, Roukis TS. Incidence of re-amputation following partial first ray amputation associated with diabetes mellitus and peripheral sensory neuropathy: a systematic review. Diabet Foot Ankle 2012. https://doi.org/10.3402/dfa.v3i0.12169.
25. Rasmussen A, Bjerre-Christensen U, Almdal TP, et al. Percutaneous flexor tenotomy for preventing and treating toe ulcers in people with diabetes mellitus. J Tissue Viability 2013. https://doi.org/10.1016/j.jtv.2013.04.001.
26. Boffeli TJ, Smith SR, Abben KW. Complete fifth ray amputation with peroneal tendon transfer to the cuboid: a review of consecutive cases involving lateral column neuropathic foot ulceration and osteomyelitis. J Foot Ankle Surg 2016. https://doi.org/10.1053/j.jfas.2016.06.005.
27. Mandolfino T, Canciglia A, Salibra M, et al. Functional outcomes of transmetatarsal amputation in the diabetic foot: timing of revascularization, wound healing and ambulatory status. Updates Surg 2016. https://doi.org/10.1007/s13304-015-0341-0.
28. Norvell DC, Turner AP, Williams RM, et al. Defining successful mobility after lower extremity amputation for complications of peripheral vascular disease and diabetes. J Vasc Surg 2011. https://doi.org/10.1016/j.jvs.2011.01.046.
29. Thomas SRYW, Perkins JMT, Magee TR, et al. Transmetatarsal amputation: an 8-year experience. Ann R Coll Surg Engl 2001;83(3):164–6.
30. Landry GJ, Silverman DA, Liem TK, et al. Predictors of healing and functional outcome following transmetatarsal amputations. Arch Surg 2011. https://doi.org/10.1001/archsurg.2011.206.
31. Stone PA, Back MR, Armstrong PA, et al. Midfoot amputations expand limb salvage rates for diabetic foot infections. Ann Vasc Surg 2005. https://doi.org/10.1007/s10016-005-7973-3.
32. Kim PJ, Steinberg JS, Kikuchi M, et al. Tibialis anterior tendon lengthening: adjunctive treatment of plantar lateral column diabetic foot ulcers. J Foot Ankle Surg 2015. https://doi.org/10.1053/j.jfas.2015.04.006.
33. DeGere MW, Grady JF. A modification of Chopart's amputation with ankle and subtalar arthrodesis by using an intramedullary nail. J Foot Ankle Surg 2005. https://doi.org/10.1053/j.jfas.2005.04.014.
34. Evans KK, Attinger CE, Al-Attar A, et al. The importance of limb preservation in the diabetic population. J Diabetes Complications 2011;25(4):227–31. https://doi.org/10.1016/j.jdiacomp.2011.02.001.
35. Schade VL. Partial or total calcanectomy as an alternative to below-the-knee amputation for limb salvage: a systematic review. J Am Podiatr Med Assoc 2012;102(5):396–405.
36. Oliver NG, Steinberg JS, Powers K, et al. Lower extremity function following partial calcanectomy in high-risk limb salvage patients. J Diabetes Res 2015. https://doi.org/10.1155/2015/432164.

Trauma in the Diabetic Limb

George T. Liu, DPM[a,b],*, Drew T. Sanders, MD[a,c],
Katherine M. Raspovic, DPM[a,b], Dane K. Wukich, MD[a,b]

KEYWORDS

- Diabetes mellitus • Orthopedic trauma • Functional outcomes
- Surgical complications

KEY POINTS

- Acute and chronic hyperglycemia lead to adverse and serious adverse events after surgery in elective and nonelective surgery.
- Poorly controlled diabetes negatively affects fracture healing.
- Comorbidities of diabetes increase risk for perioperative and short-term and long-term complications.
- Well-regulated short-term and long-term glycemic control reduces the risk of short-term and long-term complications associated with fracture surgery.

THE DIABETES EPIDEMIC

Diabetes mellitus (DM) is one of the fastest growing diseases worldwide. A pooled analysis of 751 population-based studies, representing 4.4 million patients from 146 countries, showed a significant increase in the number of adults with diabetes, from 108 million in 1980 to 422 million in 2014.[1]

In the United States, the prevalence of DM has increased from 0.93% in 1958 to 7.40% in 2015.[2–6] In 2015, approximately 9.4% of the United States population, representing an estimated 30.3 million individuals, were diagnosed with DM.[7]

Accordingly, the estimated total economic burden of DM in the United States has increased from $218 billion in 2007 to $327 billion in 2017.[8,9]

In 2017, approximately $90 billion of the indirect cost of diabetes was attributed to reduced productivity (lost wages and disability).[8] The costs of diabetes-related

Disclosures: The authors have no conflicts of financial interest related to the contents of this article.
[a] Orthopaedic Surgery, University of Texas Southwestern Medical Center, 1801 Inwood Road, Dallas, TX 75390-8883, USA; [b] Foot and Ankle Service, Orthopaedic Surgery, Parkland Memorial Hospital, Level 1 Trauma Center, 5200 Harry Hines Boulevard, Dallas, TX, 75235, USA; [c] Orthopaedic Trauma Service, Parkland Memorial Hospital, Level 1 Trauma Center, 5200 Harry Hines Boulevard, Dallas, TX 75235, USA
* Corresponding author. Department of Orthopaedic Surgery, University of Texas Southwestern Medical Center, 1801 Inwood Road, Dallas, TX 75390-8883.
E-mail address: George.liu@utsouthwestern.edu

Clin Podiatr Med Surg 36 (2019) 499–523
https://doi.org/10.1016/j.cpm.2019.02.012
0891-8422/19/© 2019 Elsevier Inc. All rights reserved.
podiatric.theclinics.com

complications has been estimated at \$47,240 per patient over a 30-year period.[10] On average, the annual costs for diabetes complications were estimated as 3 times the costs for individuals without diabetes.[11]

Patients with diabetes who undergo surgery are more likely to experience postsurgical complications and extended hospital stays compared with patients without diabetes. The hospital length of stay is estimated to be 45% longer in patients with diabetes compared with patients without diabetes.[12]

Surgical repair of diabetes-related ankle fractures is associated with significantly increased length of hospital stay, rate of in-patient postoperative complications, and rate of non-routine discharges.[13,14] Patients with diabetes typically require 1.9 days longer hospital stays and an average of \$6036 increased total charges compared with patients without diabetes.[14]

With this increasing prevalence of diabetes in both developed and developing countries, physicians and surgeons will encounter patients with diabetes regardless of their subspecialties. A retrospective study of 1166 orthopedic hospital admissions identified 385 patients with hyperglycemia (glucose level of $\geq$120 mg/dL) on admission. Only 45% of these patients had a known prior diagnosis of diabetes.[15]

LOWER EXTREMITY TRAUMA AND DIABETES

In 2007, lower extremity injuries accounted for approximately 15% of 117 million visits to emergency departments in the United States.[16] This percentage translates into approximately 17 million lower extremity injuries per year in patients with diabetes.

Sprains and strains were the most common presenting injuries (36%), followed by contusions/abrasions (19%), fractures (18%), and lacerations (8%).[17] The epidemiology of these injuries shows that an estimated 1.4 million lower extremity fractures occur in patients with diabetes each year.

Chronic hyperglycemia associated with diabetes impairs physiologic and multisystemic functions, including cellular immunity, neurologic function, and microvascular function. These physiologic derangements negatively affect the musculoskeletal system through the processes of chronic inflammation, nonenzymatic glycosylation of proteins, and oxidative stress.

DIABETES AND STATE OF INFLAMMATION

Hyperglycemia contributes to the induction of cellular stress increasing nonenzymatic glycosylation of proteins forming advanced glycation end products (AGEs), reactive oxygen species (ROS), and production of proinflammatory cytokines.[18–21]

Levels of proinflammatory cytokines, such as tumor necrosis factor (TNF)-α, interleukin (IL)-1β, IL-6, and IL-18, are increased in patients with DM, because the presence of DM seems to inhibit downregulation of inflammation once triggered.[18,22–27] This prolonged induction of inflammation potentiates increased osteoclastogenic activity, potentially resulting in impaired fracture healing and osteoporosis.[21,28,29] In addition, increased receptor activated nuclear kappa ligand (RANKL) to osteoprotegerin ratios and TNF levels both mitigate increased bone resorption activity in poorly controlled diabetes.[25,30–32]

Reduced bone formation has been shown to be related to decreased levels of osteocalcin and concomitant reduction in osteoblast formation and activity in patients with diabetes compared with patients without diabetes.[33–39] Rats with experimentally induced type 2 diabetes have lower levels of osteocalcin, bone morphogenetic proteins, and fibroblast growth factors, and reduced bone formation.[34,40,41] Inflammation seems to be a key factor because these deficits are reversed by TNF inhibition.[25,42]

Increased expression of osteoblast caspase 3 activity and Bax/Bcl-2 ratio contributes to the decreased number of osteoblasts through apoptosis.[22,43]

NORMAL PHYSIOLOGY OF FRACTURE HEALING

Fracture repair is initiated with an inflammatory response triggered by proinflammatory cytokines, such as macrophage colony-stimulating factor, TNF-α and TNF-β, IL-1, IL-6, and IL-11.[44] Both IL-1 and IL-6 are considered the most important cytokines for fracture healing. IL-1 promotes cartilaginous soft callus formation, whereas IL-6 stimulates angiogenesis through vascular endothelial growth factor production.[44,45] The acute inflammation also initiates the recruitment of mesenchymal stem cells (MSCs) and their differentiation into chondrocytes for the stage of endochondral of bone healing.[46] Endochondral tissue bridges the fracture ends and the periosteal sites during a period of 7 to 9 days to complete the soft callus stage of bone healing. Revascularization through ingrowth of blood vessels occurs through a process of apoptosis of the chondrocytes and removal of extracellular matrix, allowing angiogenic bridging across the fracture site.[47–49] Mineralization of the cartilaginous bridge provides the structural support to allow stable mechanical loading of the bone.[50–52] Conversion of soft callus to hard callus requires the differentiation of MSCs to osteoblasts and calcification of the extracellular matrix with calcium and phosphate for the formation of apatite crystals.[53–55] As the stage of hard callus formation progresses, the calcified cartilage is eventually replaced with woven bone for improved mechanical strength and rigidity. This resorption of mineralized cartilage and replacement with woven bone is mitigated by osteoclastogenesis from B-cell and T-cell production of osteoprotegerin, RANKL, TNF-α, and macrophage colony-stimulating factor.[44,56,57] The remodeling process is initiated by IL-1 and TNF-α, which stimulate osteoclastic resorption of the hard callus and replacement with lamellar bone deposition by osteoblasts.[44,58]

DIABETES AND FRACTURE HEALING

Poorly controlled diabetes adversely affects fracture healing, and patients have been reported to experience an 87% delay in fracture healing and 71% rate of malunion.[59,60] Fracture healing in animals with experimentally induced diabetes shows reduced mineralization and bony union.[61,62]

There are several stages of bone healing that are affected by diabetes. The transition from soft to hard callus formation during fracture healing is impaired by increased chondrocytes apoptosis, premature cartilage degradation, decreased osteoblast differentiation, enhanced osteoclast activity, and alteration of vascular supply.[63–66]

Advanced Glycation End Products

Increased blood glucose levels promote nonenzymatic glycosylation of proteins forming AGEs.[67–70] AGEs bind to receptors creating receptor advance glycation end products (RAGEs) which enhance expression of inflammatory cytokines.[71–73] RAGEs activate transcription factor nuclear factor-κB, which increases expression of the RANKL.[74] Although normal soft tissue and bone healing requires inflammation, the prolonged proinflammatory process observed in patients with diabetes is detrimental.

Bone remodeling and skeletal integrity are affected by nonenzymatic glycation of collagen. Increased serum glucose levels and AGEs are associated with increased formation of osteoclasts and the subsequent RAGEs formation in osteoclasts stimulates osteoclastogenesis.[75–77] RAGEs also decrease the presence of osteoprotegerin, thereby allowing increase in osteoclastogenic activity and subsequent osseous resorption.[31] AGEs concomitantly reduce osteoblast numbers by stimulating apoptosis.[78]

The structural integrity of bone is impaired by decreased enzymatic cross-links and increased nonenzymatic cross-linked collagen.[79] One cross-sectional study of 16 postmenopausal women with type II DM compared with 19 matched controls found that AGEs were associated with reduced bone material strength index by 9.2% and decreased presence of procollagen type 1.[80] Formation of AGEs have a negative impact on bone, tendon, ligament, and wound healing by decreasing fracture toughness and bone ductility, and alteration of collagen cross-linking.[81–84]

Reactive Oxygen Species

The hyperglycemic environment produces conditions for oxidative stress, which also affects bone healing. Hyperglycemia mitigates the production of ROS from superoxide production in mitochondria.[85–87] In diabetes, ROS production is stimulated by membrane-bound nicotinamide adenine dinucleotide phosphate oxidase activity, high glucose levels within mitochondria, and AGEs.[85,86,88]

Increased levels of ROS enhance the production of RAGE, RANKL, and intracellular H_2O_2, and interferes with bone healing by enhancing osteoclast formation and activity.[89–92]

Prolonged oxidative stress through the presence of ROS has been purported to affect long-term function of osteocytes and MSCs, therefore affecting bone formation, bone integrity, and remodeling activity.[90,93]

TRAUMA AND HYPERGLYCEMIC STRESS RESPONSE

Major physical trauma initiates a stress response through the sympathetic nervous system and hypothalamic-pituitary-adrenal axis known as the hypermetabolic stress response.[94,95] This response triggers release of catecholamines and glucocorticoids leading to stress carbohydrate metabolism from glycogenolysis, glucogenesis, and insulin resistance, ultimately causing hyperglycemia.[96–98]

Mild to moderate stress hyperglycemia is a compensatory survival response protecting the body from trauma and stress.[99] Increased serum glucose levels in nondiabetic patients maximize cellular glucose uptake in tissue with microvascular injury, reduces cell death from ischemia by promoting angiogenesis and inhibiting apoptosis, stimulates macrophage and neutrophil activity, and preserves neurocognitive function.[100–102]

Although stress hyperglycemia has been purported to be protective, it has also been shown to increase complications in nondiabetic orthopedic surgical patients. A prospective observational cohort single-center study of stable nondiabetic patients undergoing surgery for orthopedic injuries showed higher rates of surgical site infections (SSIs) within 30 days of index procedure in patients who had hyperglycemia compared with patients without hyperglycemia (7 out of 33, 21.2%, vs 5 out of 131, 3.8%; P = .003).[103] A retrospective study of 790 patients that underwent surgery for closed orthopedic injuries at a university-based level-I trauma center showed a 5-fold increased risk for SSI in patients with blood glucose of greater than or equal to 140 mg/dL during hospitalization.[104] A retrospective multicenter analysis of operative management of orthopedic trauma revealed a 7-fold increase risk of SSI in patients with no known history of DM who had a perioperative glucose level of greater than 220 mg/dL compared with patients less than 220 mg/dL.[105]

Stress hyperglycemia of greater than or equal to 250 mg/dL in hospitalized patients with trauma with a history of DM was associated with a 3.5-fold higher odds of mortality compared with patients with DM with normoglycemia.[106] However, patients with trauma without DM who had stress hyperglycemia during hospital admission have a 2.4-fold increased odds for mortality compared with patients with DM with diabetes-related hyperglycemia.[107]

ASSESSMENT OF TRAUMATIC INJURY IN PATIENT WITH DIABETES

The initial assessment of any patient who has sustained trauma begins with primary survey to identify any life-threatening injuries with airway, breathing, circulation, and neurologic status in accordance with the Advanced Trauma Life Support protocols.[108] Assessment of the injured limb is often performed in the secondary survey.

In general, most timelines and protocols that address orthopedic emergencies apply in patients with diabetes such as open fractures, compartment syndrome, open lacerations, joint dislocations, and polytrauma. Diabetes with acute or chronic hyperglycemia can cause both physiologic and multisystemic changes that increase morbidity in the treatment of traumatic limb injuries.

MULTIORGAN MULTISYSTEMIC INVOLVEMENT MANIFESTATIONS
Cardiovascular Disease

Diabetes is a known risk factor for cardiovascular disease and is associated with a 2-fold to 4-fold increase in cardiovascular disease (hypertension, coronary artery disease, and stroke).[109] Patients with DM who undergo surgery have a higher prevalence of CAD compared with patients without diabetes, and often their CAD is asymptomatic.[110,111]

Hyperglycemia can lead to osmotic diuresis causing hypovolemia and electrolyte imbalances. Associated tachycardia, hypomagnesemia, and hypokalemia can increase the risk of cardiac arrhythmias that contribute to perioperative cardiac-related mortality.[112]

Diabetes-associated dysfunction of the autonomic nervous system can cause cardiovascular manifestations, including resting tachycardia,[113,114] perioperative and intraoperative cardiovascular instability,[115] and arrhythmias.[116,117] Because patients with diabetes may also have concurrent peripheral neuropathy, hypercholesterolemia, and macrovascular disease, the likelihood of a silent myocardial infarction is greater.[118] The prevalence of asymptomatic myocardial infarction is estimated to be 22% in patients with DM with no known history or suspected coronary artery disease.[119]

Studies reporting postoperative mortalities in diabetic patients undergoing noncardiac surgery reported a 3% rate at 21 days and 24% rate at a median 10 months' follow-up period.[120,121]

Renal Disease

Between 2015-2016, the crude prevalence of chronic kidney disease (CKD; stages 1–4) in patients with DM is three times greater compared to patients without DM (33.4% vs 11.9%).[122]

Cardiovascular disease is the most common cause of morbidity and mortality in patients with end-stage renal disease (ESRD) and the prevalence of cardiovascular disease is estimated to be 50% in patients requiring dialysis.[123–127]

Mortalities at 10-year follow-up of patients admitted for major inpatient surgery for all surgical specialties were 6%, 19%, and 27% for patients with no kidney disease, acute kidney injury with CKD, and ESRD, respectively ($P<.001$).[128]

Electrolyte imbalances may be present in patients with CKD (both ESRD and non-ESRD) who need surgery. If patients have both hyperkalemia and fluid overload, urgent preoperative dialysis may be indicated.[126]

Platelet dysfunction caused by uremic toxin increases the risk of perioperative bleeding.[129,130] Patients with CKD often are anemic because of decreased renal production of erythropoietin. Consequently, preoperative and postoperative blood transfusion may be needed to maintain a hemoglobin level greater than or equal to 7 to 8 g/dL in patients with stable cardiovascular disease undergoing lower-risk musculoskeletal surgery or a symptomatic patients with hemoglobin level less than 10 g/dL to address hemodynamic instability and/or ischemic myocardial symptoms.[131]

Peripheral Arterial Disease

The prevalence of peripheral arterial disease (PAD), defined as an ankle-brachial index (ABI) less than 0.90, in patients with DM was estimated at between 33% and 42%.[132,133]

The long-term glycemic control has been shown to be an independent risk factor for PAD in patients with diabetes, because every 1% increase in glycosylated hemoglobin increases the risk of PAD by 28%.[134]

In patients with manifestations of diabetic foot disease (infection, skin ulcers, neuropathic arthropathy) the prevalence of PAD has been reported to be as high as 50%.[135,136]

The clinical assessment of arterial flow in the setting of lower extremity trauma may be difficult because of pain, swelling, or degree of injury to the limb. With long-standing DM, presence or absence of palpable pulses may not be a reliable indicator of blood flow. Although the absence of pedal pulse was associated with a 4.9-fold likelihood of PAD, the presence of a palpable pulse did not exclude the diagnosis of PAD.[137,138] In addition, manifestations of nonocclusive medial arterial calcinosis with long-standing DM may render the artery noncompressible.[139] Hand-held Dopplers may be used to evaluate amplitude and phasic waveforms to the dorsalis pedis and posterior tibial and popliteal arteries. Noninvasive vascular studies with bilateral measurements of the ABI, toe-brachial index, absolute great toe pressures, and waveforms are the primary standard to evaluate arterial flow; however, they may not be feasible in patients with DM with lower extremity trauma.

If severe vascular compromise is suspected clinically, computed tomographic angiogram or lower extremity arteriogram along with vascular surgery service consultation may be indicated.

Diabetic Neuropathy

Neuropathies are the most common long-term complications of DM. Distal symmetric polyneuropathy (DSPN) and diabetic autonomic neuropathies can be the source of complications through impaired sensory and sympathetic and parasympathetic function of the nervous system.[140–142]

The overall prevalence of DSPN was reported to be 28.5% of 6487 patients with diabetes in one multicenter study and increased as the duration of DM increased (20.8% of patients with diabetes for <5 years and 36.8% of patients with diabetes for >10 years).[143] One study reported the prevalence of DSPN in patients with DM undergoing lower extremity surgery as high as 77.2% (304 of 394 patients).[144]

Diagnosing DSPN can be done through several objective methods, such as monofilament examination, vibration testing, or ankle reflex examination. Peripheral neuropathy can be inferred if diabetic patients ambulate on an injured limb without complaint of pain. The Michigan Neuropathy Screening Index is a validated screening tool that uses a 5.07 (10 g) Semmes-Weinstein monofilament, vibratory sensation with a 128-Hz tuning fork, evaluation of gastrocnemius-soleus muscle stretch reflex, identification of ulceration, and presence of foot deformities.[145]

The lack of protective response is the critical factor that leads to complications seen with DSPN because patients with trauma are often unaware of the severity of musculoskeletal injury. Neuropathic patients often continue to ambulate on a potentially unstable joint or bony injuries, creating an ongoing inflammatory environment of injury that can lead to skin compromise, malunion, and/or Charcot neuroarthropathy (CN). In patients with CN, only 36% of patients with DM reported some form of trauma and 12% reported foot surgery in the preceding 6 months.[146]

Neuropathy is an essential component for the pathogenesis of CN with sensory neuropathy, dysfunction of the autonomic nervous system, altering arterial perfusion, triggering cellular inflammation, and increasing bony turnover.[147–150]

Peripheral neuropathy may affect skeletal homeostasis and mineral metabolism. Patients with DM and severe peripheral neuropathy showed significant lower bone mineral density compared with control subjects.[151] Innervation of the skeletal system with adrenergic and peptidergic nerve terminals suggests a role of neural mediation of bone remodeling with neuropeptides.[152,153] Calcitonin gene–related peptide (CGRP) is a neuropeptide found in small myelinated A-δ type and unmyelinated C-type fibers and has been shown to modulate the integrity of trabecular bone.[154] Studies have shown the association between absence of CGRP and osteopenia from reduced osteoblast activity but also though a direct action on osteoclasts.[155,156] Bone biopsies in patients with diabetic peripheral neuropathy and CN showed decrease of CGRP expression compared with patients with DM without peripheral neuropathy.[157] These findings are consistent with clinical reports of lower bone mineral density seen in patients with DM with CN.[29,158,159]

The presence of peripheral neuropathy is a predictive factor for SSI. Although diabetes is the leading cause of peripheral neuropathy, neuropathy alone has been identified as an independent risk factor associated with a more than 4-fold increase for SSI.[160–162] Although the specific relationship between infectious complications and neuropathy is not clearly elucidated, autonomic nerve dysfunction and impaired microcirculatory response to injury or inflammation have been purported to contribute to the host tissue vulnerability to infection.[163] In addition, patients with peripheral neuropathy have reduced release of neuropeptides, which are mediators of angiogenesis, cellular immunity, and inflammatory healing response.[164–166]

Vitamin D Deficiencies

Vitamin D deficiencies are prevalent among patients in the United States. The Endocrine Society defines a vitamin D deficiency as a 25-hydroxyvitamin D [25(OH)D] level less than 20 ng/mL and vitamin D insufficiency as a 25(OH)D level of 21 to 29 ng/mL.[167] A National Health and Nutrition Examination Survey conducted between 2005 and 2006 reported an overall prevalence of vitamin D levels in to be 41.6% of 4495 participants.[168] A survey of vitamin D levels from 1119 consecutive orthopedic surgery patients reported deficiency as a mean of 20.6 ng/mL.[169] A survey of 889 patients with orthopedic trauma treated for acute fractures revealed an overall prevalence of vitamin D deficiency/insufficiency of 77%, whereas the prevalence of vitamin D deficiency alone was 39%.[170]

Vitamin D deficiencies have been reported to be significantly less common in patients with DM compared with patients without DM.[171]

Deficiencies in vitamin D can lead to lower calcium absorption from the intestine and hypocalcemia. Lower serum calcium level stimulates parathyroid hormone secretion, thereby depleting calcium from bones. Although the optimal vitamin D level for bone healing has not been established, 25(OH)D level of greater than 20 ng/mL is considered necessary to maintain skeletal health. Deficiencies in vitamin D have been implicated in nonhealing of bone. One retrospective study reported 68% vitamin D deficiency in 23% of patients with tibial nonunions.[172] Higher vitamin D levels have been associated with improved functional outcomes and lower risk of falls after hip fracture surgery compared with patients who were vitamin D deficient.[173,174]

Robertson and colleagues[175] evaluated the effectiveness of a vitamin D treatment protocol to address low serum vitamin D levels in 201 patients with orthopedic trauma. All patients were instructed to start over-the-counter vitamin D_3 1000 IU and 1500 mg of calcium per day. Patients with vitamin D deficiency/insufficiency received 50,000 IU of ergocalciferol (D_2) weekly until the 25(OH)D level was normalized or fracture healed. Of 88 patients who were identified as vitamin D insufficient, 54.5% improved to normal and, of the 81 patients who were vitamin D deficient, 74% improved to insufficient. The increases of vitamin D levels in both groups were statistically significant.

Perioperative Glycemic Control

Perioperative hyperglycemia adversely increases postsurgical morbidity and mortality in cardiac, orthopedic, and general surgery.[103,176–179] Hyperglycemia in DM has been shown to impair host immunity by decreasing chemotaxis of leukocytes, phagocytosis, and intracellular bactericidal activity.[180,181]

Perioperative hyperglycemia is a known risk factor for SSI in patients undergoing orthopedic surgery with and without diabetes.[103,104,160,182,183] Approximately 12% of patients with DM who underwent foot and ankle surgery with serum glucose levels greater than or equal to 200 mg/dL during the admission developed an SSI compared with 5.2% of patients whose serum glucose level never exceeded 200 mg/dL ($P = .03$).[183]

Long-term Glycemic Control

Glycated hemoglobin A1c (HbA1c) is created through irreversible glycation of the N-terminal valine residue of each β chain of hemoglobin A and reflects glycemic control over the previous 2 to 3 months. Since 1988, HbA1c has been the recommended serologic study by the American Diabetes Association for routine monitoring of patients with DM.[184] Although the goals is not to manage HbA1c in the trauma setting, glycated hemoglobin provides a good indication of a patient's long-term glycemic control and should be used to assist in DM management in the postoperative period and for discharge planning.

Increased HbA1c level is a known risk factor for complications following orthopedic and nonorthopedic surgery in patients with and without diabetes.[160,162,185–193]

Domek and colleagues[186] reported that every 1% increase in HbA1c was associated with 5% increased odds of developing a complication after foot and ankle surgery.

The American Diabetes Association has considered a target HbA1c of less than 7% as reasonable glycemic control based on the associated reduction of microvascular complications associated with diabetes.[194] Although this target HbA1c level was not based on surgical outcomes, HbA1c of less than 7% has been the recommended level for the decision to proceed with elective surgery.

The association between HbA1c and surgical complications has been reported. Jupiter and colleagues[191] reported that the mean HbA1c level of patients with DM that experienced a postoperative infection was 8.3% $\pm$ 1.9% compared with 7.2% $\pm$ 1.4% without infection ($P<.001$). Wukich and colleagues[160] found that the SSI rate was 2.5 times higher in patients with a HbA1c level greater than 8% compared with less than 8%. Shibuya and colleagues[195] showed significantly higher rates of malunions, delayed unions, and nonunions in foot and ankle surgery in patients with DM with HbA1c levels greater than 7%.

MANAGEMENT OF HYPERGLYCEMIA

Perioperative management of hyperglycemia in patients with trauma with diabetes can reduce the relative risk of immediate postsurgical complications. A retrospective study of patients with DM undergoing coronary artery bypass grafting surgery reported significant reduction in SSI (1.5% vs 3.5%; P = .001) in patients that had tight perioperative glycemic control of 80 mg/dL to 110 mg/dL compared with routine control in the perioperative period.[196] A randomized multicenter trial, showed lower rates of postoperative complications (24.3% vs 8.6%), including wound infection, bacteremia, pneumonia, and respiratory and acute renal failure in patients with DM undergoing general surgery with basal-bolus insulin compared with sliding-scale insulin (145 ± 32 mg/dL vs 172 ± 47 mg/dL).[197]

Although there are no randomized controlled trials evaluating the role of glycemic management in patients with DM undergoing orthopedic surgery, one retrospective observational study reported a reduction of SSI rates in patients undergoing hip and knee replacement surgery through an evidence-based perioperative glucose monitoring algorithm.[198]

Preoperative random glucose and HbA1c levels establish current and long-term hyperglycemic control. Although hyperglycemia in patients with trauma should not necessarily delay emergent or urgent surgical intervention, management of hyperglycemia may begin concurrently.

Although there is no evidence-based target perioperative glycemic index in patients with orthopedic trauma, there are established glycemic target end points for inpatient care. Tight glycemic control of 80 to 110 mg/dL with intensive insulin therapy was found to significantly reduce in-hospital mortality and morbidity in intensive care patients.[199] The Normoglycemia in Intensive Care Evaluation and Surviving Using Glucose Algorithm Regulation (NICE-SUGAR) multinational, randomized trial evaluating intensive glucose control (81–108 mg/dL) compared with conventional glucose control (≤180 mg/dL) in intensive care patients reported significant rates of severe hypoglycemia (≤40 mg/dL) in the intensive glucose control group compared with the conventional glucose control group (6.8% vs 0.5%; P<.001) and absolute increase in mortality at 90 days (27.5% vs 24.9%; P = .02).[200] A consensus statement issued by the American Association of Clinical Endocrinologists and the American Diabetes Association has since recommended glucose targets between 140 and 180 mg/dL with intravenous insulin in critically ill patients and less than 140 mg/dL in non–critically ill patients.[12] Insulin regimen should be reassessed if blood glucose level decreases to less than 100 mg/dL to avoid hypoglycemia and should be modified in patients who decrease to less than 70 mg/dL.

Although there is no evidence-based standard to guide cancellation of surgery because of hyperglycemia, in general, surgery should be postponed if blood glucose level is greater than 400 mg/dL or if the patient is in a compromised metabolic state, such as diabetic ketoacidosis or hyperglycemic hyperosmolar syndrome.[201]

One study of glycemic management in patients with DM undergoing total knee or hip arthroplasty recommended monitoring blood glucose in the preoperative, intraoperative, and postoperative phases of the surgical encounter to reduce SSI rates.[198] For inpatients, blood glucose monitoring is recommended 4 times daily. Intravenous insulin continues to be the appropriate method for glycemic control for hospitalized patients. The use of a sliding-scale insulin regimen alone is not recommended based on several studies showing short-acting insulin to be ineffective in managing hyperglycemia in the inpatient setting because of the absence of a basal insulin component of therapy.[202–206] If a patient has 2 or more blood glucose levels greater than 200 mg/dL, consult to a hospitalist and/or endocrinologist is recommended to assume glycemic management. Patients' blood glucose levels should be stabilized, treatment regimen established, outpatient DM management strategies provided, and immediate follow-up with their primary care physicians or endocrinologists before patient discharge from the hospital to ensure continued glycemic control.[207]

DIABETES, SURGERY, AND QUALITY ASSURANCE METRICS

Patient safety metrics are monitored and publicly reported by the Centers for Medicare & Medicaid Services in an effort to reduce costly unplanned readmission, reoperation, length of hospital stay, and mortality. Hyperglycemia and presence of DM-related comorbidities negatively affect postoperative outcomes in musculoskeletal surgery. Adverse events, such as venous thromboembolic events, SSIs, and complications of implants or grafts, are among the quality metrics that are reported for musculoskeletal surgery.

Preadmission hyperglycemia with increased HbA1c level was found to be an independent risk factor for pulmonary embolism (PE) and increased hospital length of stay. A retrospective review of medical records of patients undergoing major orthopedic surgery identified an incidence of PE of 1.5%. A preoperative glucose level greater than or equal to 200 mg/dL independently increased risk for a symptomatic PE by a factor of 3 ($P = .015$) compared with patients with preoperative glucose level of less than 110 mg/dL.[208]

One study reported a poor postoperative recovery rate of less than 50% for cervical laminoplasty for cervical spondylotic myelopathy in patients with DM with HgA1c level greater than or equal to 6.5% (odds ratio, 2.591; $P = .0193$) and greater than or equal to 10 years' duration of DM (odds ratio, 2.245; $P = .0321$).[209]

A retrospective analysis of 13,272 patients undergoing primary joint arthroplasty in the Veterans Administration health care system, reported that 38% of patients had an increased perioperative HbA1c level greater than or equal to 7%, which carried an increased risk of mortality (hazard ratio, 1.3; $P = .01$).[210]

Significant increases in hospital stays, postoperative complications, and nonroutine discharges are common in patients with DM who undergo operative management for unstable ankle fractures.[13,14] Specifically, patients with DM often incur 1.9 days additional hospital stay and $6036 increased total hospital charges compared with patients without DM.[14]

SooHoo and colleagues[211] compared complication rates following open reduction with internal fixation of ankle fractures between 4710 patients with uncomplicated and complicated diabetes from a statewide discharge database. Complicated DM was defined as the presence of end-organ damage associated with DM disease. They reported an increased 90-day unplanned reoperation rate of 4.4% in patients with complicated DM compared with 1.4% in patients with uncomplicated DM. In addition, 90-day mortalities following operatively managed ankle fractures in patients with complicated DM were higher (4.3%) compared with patients with uncomplicated DM (2.5%).

OUTCOMES IN LOWER EXTREMITY TRAUMA WITH DIABETES

There is a paucity of studies that compare adverse outcomes between patients with and without DM that undergo surgery for lower extremity fractures. A systematic review identifying 8 studies evaluating healing outcomes of lower extremity fractures in patients with and without DM reported a 7.3-fold increase in the odds for nonunion in patients with DM.[212]

Tibia Fractures

Aderinto and Keating[213] reported outcomes of intramedullary nailing of tibial fractures in 20 patients with DM compared with 20 patients without DM. For the closed injuries, delayed union was seen after 6 months in 52% of the patients with DM compared with 43% of patients without DM. Exchange tibial nailing was required in 9% of the closed fractures in the patients with DM and none for the patients without DM. Increased rate of SSIs occurred in patients with DM compared with the patients without DM (17% vs 9%; $P = .489$).

Tibial Pilon Fractures

Kline and colleagues[214] performed a retrospective review of outcomes following surgically managed intraarticular distal tibial fractures between patients with and without DM. At a minimum of 6 months' follow up, 14 fractures in 13 patients with DM, and 69 fractures in 68 without DM, were evaluated. Although the wound complication rate was 7% for both patient groups, there was a significant increase in overall infection rate of 71% (19% superficial and 43% deep) in patients with DM compared with 19% (10% superficial and 9% deep) in patients without DM. The overall odds for infectious complications were 10.7-fold for patients with DM that underwent surgical management for pilon fractures. The rate of nonunion/delayed union was 43% in the DM group compared with 16% in the non-DM group. The overall increased odds for nonunion was 3.95-fold for patients with DM that underwent surgical management for pilon fractures.

Ankle Fractures

McCormack and Leith[60] performed a case-controlled comparison of displaced malleolar fracture management in 26 patients with DM with a matched group of patients without DM. The complication rate of the 19 patients with ankle fractures treated operatively was 42.3%, including short-term complications of wound necrosis, deep SSI malunion, and late complications of amputation followed by death. Diabetic ankle fractures treated nonoperatively had a 71.4% malunion rate. No complications were seen in ankle fractures managed in the matched patient group without DM.

Blotter and colleagues[215] conducted a retrospective analysis of operatively managed ankle fractures in 21 patients with DM (7 insulin-dependent DM and 14 non–insulin-dependent DM) compared with 46 patients without DM matched for sex, age, and fracture severity. The complication rate in the patient group with DM was 43% with 13 complications in 9 patients, including 5 deep and 2 superficial infections, 3 hardware failures, 1 plantar ulcer, 1 wound complication, and 1 case of complex regional pain syndrome. Seven additional operative procedures were required in the DM group, including 2 below-knee amputations. Rate of complications seen in the non-DM group was 15.5%. The relative risk for complications in patients with DM that underwent operative management of ankle fractures was 2.76 times higher compared with the control group.

Flynn and colleagues[216] compared complications between 73 nondiabetic and 25 diabetic patients with closed ankle fractures treated both operatively and nonoperatively. The overall risk of infection in operatively treated ankle fractures was approximately 3 times greater in patients with DM (26.3%) compared with patients without

DM (8.8%). Patients with DM with ankle fractures treated with cast immobilization had a greater tendency for infection from wounds or ulcers (16%) compared with no infections seen in patients without DM treated in the same fashion.

Jones and colleagues[217] retrospectively performed an age-matched, gender-matched, and fracture type–matched comparison of complication rates of closed, rotational ankle fractures with operative versus nonoperative treatment between 3 groups: 21 patients with DM with comorbidities, 21 patients with DM without comorbidities, and 42 patients without DM. Comorbidities were defined as the presence of peripheral neuropathy, nephropathy, retinopathy, or arterial disease (peripheral or coronary); history of CN; or history of major amputation. Complications of treatment were identified as infection requiring antibiotics, recurrent ulceration, unplanned return to the operating room, malunion, nonunion, continued bracing at 6 months, development of CN of the ankle, transtibial amputation, and mortality. Patients with DM without comorbidities had almost equivalent complication rates to their controls. Patients with DM and comorbidities were 5.45 times more likely to experience complications compared with matched controls (47% vs 14%; $P = .034$).

Guo and colleagues[218] reported on 12-month functional outcomes of operatively managed ankle fractures between matched cohorts of 36 patients with preoperatively neglected type 2 DM and 36 patients without DM. Of the patients with newly diagnosed DM, 27 were placed on oral hypoglycemic medications and 5 were placed on insulin postoperatively. Open reduction and internal fixation was performed within 6 hours of injury for both groups. Although higher rates of SSI were seen in the DM group compared with the non-DM controls (13% vs 5%), this difference was not statistically significant and did not affect the final outcome because both groups showed similar functional outcome ankle scores at 12 months. Surgeons should recognize that this study was underpowered to detect a statistically significant difference because the post hoc power analysis of this study was only 21.7%. Assuming a 1-to-1 enrollment, 200 subjects in each arm of this study would be necessary to achieve 80% power.

Wukich and colleagues[138] evaluated the role of diabetes-related comorbidities in ankle fracture surgery outcomes. They retrospectively compared the complication rates of ankle fracture surgery between 46 patients with complicated diabetes (manifestations of peripheral neuropathy, nephropathy, and/or PAD) and 59 patients with uncomplicated diabetes (no manifestations of diabetes-related comorbidities). Comparing complicated versus uncomplicated diabetes, patients with complicated diabetes that underwent ankle fracture surgery had 3.8 times higher risk of overall complications (50% vs 22.8%); 3.4 times higher risk for noninfectious complication, such as malunion, nonunion, or CN (28.9% vs 11.9%); and a 5 times higher risk of requiring revision surgery (26.7% vs 6.8%).

SUMMARY AND EVIDENCE-BASED RECOMMENDATIONS
Hyperglycemia and Bone Healing

Hyperglycemia affects bone healing through increased production of proinflammatory cytokines and formation of AGE and ROS, which promote osteoclastogenesis and decreases osteoblastic activity.

Hyperglycemia and Complications

Hyperglycemia is a risk factor for all-cause complications in patients both with and without DM.

Diabetes and Comorbidities

Multisystemic comorbid manifestations of DM can increase risk of short-term and long-term surgical morbidity and mortality.

Optimal Preoperative Glycemic Control

Although there is no evidence-based recommendation on optimal perioperative glycemic level in patients with orthopedic trauma undergoing surgery, the American Association of Clinical Endocrinologists and the American Diabetes Association recommend glucose targets between 140 and 180 mg/dL with intravenous insulin in critically ill patients and less than 140 mg/dL in non–critically ill patients. Hypoglycemia should be avoided.

Optimal Preoperative Hemoglobin A1c Level

A preoperative HbA1c level of less than 7% has been associated with lower risk of perioperative adverse events and long-term postoperative complications. Glycated hemoglobin provides an index of the patient's long-term glycemic control and should be used to assist in DM management in the postoperative period and for discharge planning.

Optimal Postoperative Glycemic Control

Intravenous insulin is the best method of glycemic control for hospitalized patients. Use of sliding-scale insulin alone is ineffective in managing hyperglycemia in the inpatient setting. Optimal perioperative glycemic management is best achieved when comanagement of the patient is the responsibility of both the surgeon and a medical consultant (hospitalist, endocrinologist, or primary care physician experienced in inpatient care).

Vitamin D Deficiencies

Identifying vitamin D deficiencies/insufficiencies preoperatively may assist in assessing risk factors that may negatively affect bone healing and overall skeletal homeostasis. Referral to a primary care physician or endocrinologist to establish a dietary and supplementation regimen to restore vitamin D to therapeutic levels is recommended.

Postoperative Discharge Planning

Coordination of discharge planning is critical in reducing complications and the rate of readmission. Follow-up with the patient's primary care physician or endocrinologist is necessary to continue optimal management of the patient's glucose control while at home or in the skilled nursing facility.

REFERENCES

1. NCD Risk Factor Collaboration (NCD-RisC). Worldwide trends in diabetes since 1980: a pooled analysis of 751 population-based studies with 4.4 million participants. Lancet 2016;387(10027):1513–30.

2. Harris MI. Prevalence of noninsulin-dependent diabetes and impaired glucose tolerance. In: Harris MI, Hamman RF, editors. Diabetes in America. National Institutes of Health; 1985.

3. Massey JT, Moore TF, Parsons VL, et al. Design and estimation for the national health interview survey, 1985–994. Hyattsville (MD): National Center for Health Statistics. Vital and Health Statistics 1989;2(110).

4. Botman SL, Moore TF, Moriarity CL, et al. Design and estimation for the national Health interview survey, 1995–2004. National Center for Health Statistics. Vital and Health Statistics 2000;2(130).

5. Geiss LS, Wang J, Cheng YJ, et al. Prevalence and incidence trends for diagnosed diabetes among adults aged 20 to 79 years, United States, 1980-2012. JAMA 2014;312(12):1218–26.

6. Parsons VL, Moriarity C, Jonas K, et al. Design and estimation for the national health interview survey, 2006-2015. Vital Health Stat 2 2014;(165):1–53.

7. Centers for Disease Control and Prevention. National Diabetes Statistics Report, 2017. Atlanta (GA): Centers for Disease Control and Prevention, U.S. Dept of Health and Human Services; 2017.

8. American Diabetes Association. Economic costs of diabetes in the U.S. In 2017. Diabetes Care 2018;41(5):917–28.

9. Dall TM, Zhang Y, Chen YJ, et al. The economic burden of diabetes. Health Aff (Millwood) 2010;29(2):297–303.

10. Caro JJ, Ward AJ, O'Brien JA. Lifetime costs of complications resulting from type 2 diabetes in the U.S. Diabetes Care 2002;25(3):476–81.

11. Vojta D, De Sa J, Prospect T, et al. Effective interventions for stemming the growing crisis of diabetes and prediabetes: a national payer's perspective. Health Aff (Millwood) 2012;31(1):20–6.

12. Moghissi ES, Korytkowski MT, DiNardo M, et al. American Association of Clinical Endocrinologists and American Diabetes Association consensus statement on inpatient glycemic control. Endocr Pract 2009;15(4):353–69.

13. Ganesh SP, Pietrobon R, Cecilio WA, et al. The impact of diabetes on patient outcomes after ankle fracture. J Bone Joint Surg Am 2005;87(8):1712–8.

14. Regan DK, Manoli A 3rd, Hutzler L, et al. Impact of diabetes mellitus on surgical quality measures after ankle fracture surgery: implications for "Value-Based" compensation and "pay for performance". J Orthop Trauma 2015;29(12): e483–6.

15. Cohen GD, Schnall SB, Holtom P. New onset diabetes mellitus in patients presenting with extremity infections. Clin Orthop Relat Res 2002;(403):45–8.

16. Niska R, Bhuiya F, Xu J. National hospital ambulatory medical care survey: 2007 emergency department summary. Natl Health Stat Report 2010;(26):1–31.

17. Lambers K, Ootes D, Ring D. Incidence of patients with lower extremity injuries presenting to US emergency departments by anatomic region, disease category, and age. Clin Orthop Relat Res 2012;470(1):284–90.

18. Graves DT, Kayal RA. Diabetic complications and dysregulated innate immunity. Front Biosci 2008;13:1227–39.

19. Moseley KF. Type 2 diabetes and bone fractures. Curr Opin Endocrinol Diabetes Obes 2012;19(2):128–35.

20. Weinberg E, Maymon T, Weinreb M. AGEs induce caspase-mediated apoptosis of rat BMSCs via TNFalpha production and oxidative stress. J Mol Endocrinol 2014;52(1):67–76.

21. Yamagishi S. Role of advanced glycation end products (AGEs) in osteoporosis in diabetes. Curr Drug Targets 2011;12(14):2096–102.

22. Andriankaja OM, Galicia J, Dong G, et al. Gene expression dynamics during diabetic periodontitis. J Dent Res 2012;91(12):1160–5.

23. Devaraj S, Cheung AT, Jialal I, et al. Evidence of increased inflammation and microcirculatory abnormalities in patients with type 1 diabetes and their role in microvascular complications. Diabetes 2007;56(11):2790–6.

24. Hatanaka E, Monteagudo PT, Marrocos MS, et al. Neutrophils and monocytes as potentially important sources of proinflammatory cytokines in diabetes. Clin Exp Immunol 2006;146(3):443–7.

25. Pacios S, Kang J, Galicia J, et al. Diabetes aggravates periodontitis by limiting repair through enhanced inflammation. FASEB J 2012;26(4):1423–30.

26. Pradhan AD, Manson JE, Rifai N, et al. C-reactive protein, interleukin 6, and risk of developing type 2 diabetes mellitus. JAMA 2001;286(3):327–34.

27. Vozarova B, Weyer C, Lindsay RS, et al. High white blood cell count is associated with a worsening of insulin sensitivity and predicts the development of type 2 diabetes. Diabetes 2002;51(2):455–61.

28. Alblowi J, Tian C, Siqueira MF, et al. Chemokine expression is upregulated in chondrocytes in diabetic fracture healing. Bone 2013;53(1):294–300.

29. Krakauer JC, McKenna MJ, Buderer NF, et al. Bone loss and bone turnover in diabetes. Diabetes 1995;44(7):775–82.

30. Mahamed DA, Marleau A, Alnaeeli M, et al. G(-) anaerobes-reactive CD4+ T-cells trigger RANKL-mediated enhanced alveolar bone loss in diabetic NOD mice. Diabetes 2005;54(5):1477–86.

31. Santos VR, Lima JA, Goncalves TE, et al. Receptor activator of nuclear factor-kappa B ligand/osteoprotegerin ratio in sites of chronic periodontitis of subjects with poorly and well-controlled type 2 diabetes. J Periodontol 2010;81(10): 1455–65.

32. Sassi F, Buondonno I, Luppi C, et al. Type 2 diabetes affects bone cells precursors and bone turnover. BMC Endocr Disord 2018;18(1):55.

33. Bouillon R. Diabetic bone disease. Low turnover osteoporosis related to decreased IGF-I production. Verh K Acad Geneeskd Belg 1992;54(4):365–91 [discussion: 391–2].

34. Bouillon R, Bex M, Van Herck E, et al. Influence of age, sex, and insulin on osteoblast function: osteoblast dysfunction in diabetes mellitus. J Clin Endocrinol Metab 1995;80(4):1194–202.

35. Lumachi F, Camozzi V, Tombolan V, et al. Bone mineral density, osteocalcin, and bone-specific alkaline phosphatase in patients with insulin-dependent diabetes mellitus. Ann N Y Acad Sci 2009;1173(Suppl 1):E64–7.

36. Maddaloni E, D'Onofrio L, Lauria A, et al. Osteocalcin levels are inversely associated with Hba1c and BMI in adult subjects with long-standing type 1 diabetes. J Endocrinol Invest 2014;37(7):661–6.

37. Sarkar PD, Choudhury AB. Relationships between serum osteocalcin levels versus blood glucose, insulin resistance and markers of systemic inflammation in central Indian type 2 diabetic patients. Eur Rev Med Pharmacol Sci 2013; 17(12):1631–5.

38. Masse PG, Pacifique MB, Tranchant CC, et al. Bone metabolic abnormalities associated with well-controlled type 1 diabetes (IDDM) in young adult women: a disease complication often ignored or neglected. J Am Coll Nutr 2010; 29(4):419–29.

39. Peng J, Hui K, Hao C, et al. Low bone turnover and reduced angiogenesis in streptozotocin-induced osteoporotic mice. Connect Tissue Res 2016;57(4): 277–89.

40. Horcajada-Molteni MN, Chanteranne B, Lebecque P, et al. Amylin and bone metabolism in streptozotocin-induced diabetic rats. J Bone Miner Res 2001; 16(5):958–65.

41. Verhaeghe J, Van Herck E, van Bree R, et al. Decreased osteoblast activity in spontaneously diabetic rats. In vivo studies on the pathogenesis. Endocrine 1997;7(2):165–75.

42. Pacios S, Andriankaja O, Kang J, et al. Bacterial infection increases periodontal bone loss in diabetic rats through enhanced apoptosis. Am J Pathol 2013; 183(6):1928–35.

43. Coe LM, Irwin R, Lippner D, et al. The bone marrow microenvironment contributes to type I diabetes induced osteoblast death. J Cell Physiol 2011;226(2): 477–83.

44. Kon T, Cho TJ, Aizawa T, et al. Expression of osteoprotegerin, receptor activator of NF-kappaB ligand (osteoprotegerin ligand) and related proinflammatory cytokines during fracture healing. J Bone Miner Res 2001;16(6):1004–14.

45. Yang X, Ricciardi BF, Hernandez-Soria A, et al. Callus mineralization and maturation are delayed during fracture healing in interleukin-6 knockout mice. Bone 2007;41(6):928–36.

46. Granero-Molto F, Weis JA, Miga MI, et al. Regenerative effects of transplanted mesenchymal stem cells in fracture healing. Stem Cells 2009;27(8):1887–98.

47. Lee FY, Choi YW, Behrens FF, et al. Programmed removal of chondrocytes during endochondral fracture healing. J Orthop Res 1998;16(1):144–50.

48. Lehmann W, Edgar CM, Wang K, et al. Tumor necrosis factor alpha (TNF-alpha) coordinately regulates the expression of specific matrix metalloproteinases (MMPS) and angiogenic factors during fracture healing. Bone 2005;36(2): 300–10.

49. Li G, White G, Connolly C, et al. Cell proliferation and apoptosis during fracture healing. J Bone Miner Res 2002;17(5):791–9.

50. Gerstenfeld LC, Alkhiary YM, Krall EA, et al. Three-dimensional reconstruction of fracture callus morphogenesis. J Histochem Cytochem 2006;54(11):1215–28.

51. Richardson JB, Cunningham JL, Goodship AE, et al. Measuring stiffness can define healing of tibial fractures. J Bone Joint Surg Br 1994;76(3):389–94.

52. Wade RH, Moorcroft CI, Thomas PB. Fracture stiffness as a guide to the management of tibial fractures. J Bone Joint Surg Br 2001;83(4):533–5.

53. French DM, Kaul RJ, D'Souza AL, et al. WISP-1 is an osteoblastic regulator expressed during skeletal development and fracture repair. Am J Pathol 2004; 165(3):855–67.

54. Zhong N, Gersch RP, Hadjiargyrou M. Wnt signaling activation during bone regeneration and the role of Dishevelled in chondrocyte proliferation and differentiation. Bone 2006;39(1):5–16.

55. Ketenjian AY, Arsenis C. Morphological and biochemical studies during differentiation and calcification of fracture callus cartilage. Clin Orthop Relat Res 1975; 107:266–73.

56. Gerstenfeld LC, Cho TJ, Kon T, et al. Impaired intramembranous bone formation during bone repair in the absence of tumor necrosis factor-alpha signaling. Cells Tissues Organs 2001;169(3):285–94.

57. Konnecke I, Serra A, El Khassawna T, et al. T and B cells participate in bone repair by infiltrating the fracture callus in a two-wave fashion. Bone 2014;64: 155–65.

58. Balga R, Wetterwald A, Portenier J, et al. Tumor necrosis factor-alpha: alternative role as an inhibitor of osteoclast formation in vitro. Bone 2006;39(2):325–35.

59. Loder RT. The influence of diabetes mellitus on the healing of closed fractures. Clin Orthop Relat Res 1988;(232):210–6.

60. McCormack RG, Leith JM. Ankle fractures in diabetics. Complications of surgical management. J Bone Joint Surg Br 1998;80(4):689–92.
61. Follak N, Kloting I, Merk H. Influence of diabetic metabolic state on fracture healing in spontaneously diabetic rats. Diabetes Metab Res Rev 2005;21(3):288–96.
62. Funk JR, Hale JE, Carmines D, et al. Biomechanical evaluation of early fracture healing in normal and diabetic rats. J Orthop Res 2000;18(1):126–32.
63. Bacevic M, Brkovic B, Albert A, et al. Does oxidative stress play a role in altered characteristics of diabetic bone? A systematic review. Calcif Tissue Int 2017; 101(6):553–63.
64. Kayal RA, Siqueira M, Alblowi J, et al. TNF-alpha mediates diabetes-enhanced chondrocyte apoptosis during fracture healing and stimulates chondrocyte apoptosis through FOXO1. J Bone Miner Res 2010;25(7):1604–15.
65. Stolzing A, Sellers D, Llewelyn O, et al. Diabetes induced changes in rat mesenchymal stem cells. Cells Tissues Organs 2010;191(6):453–65.
66. Tuominen JT, Impivaara O, Puukka P, et al. Bone mineral density in patients with type 1 and type 2 diabetes. Diabetes Care 1999;22(7):1196–200.
67. Charonis AS, Reger LA, Dege JE, et al. Laminin alterations after in vitro nonenzymatic glycosylation. Diabetes 1990;39(7):807–14.
68. Tanaka S, Avigad G, Brodsky B, et al. Glycation induces expansion of the molecular packing of collagen. J Mol Biol 1988;203(2):495–505.
69. Tsilibary EC, Charonis AS, Reger LA, et al. The effect of nonenzymatic glucosylation on the binding of the main noncollagenous NC1 domain to type IV collagen. J Biol Chem 1988;263(9):4302–8.
70. Wells-Knecht KJ, Zyzak DV, Litchfield JE, et al. Mechanism of autoxidative glycosylation: identification of glyoxal and arabinose as intermediates in the autoxidative modification of proteins by glucose. Biochemistry 1995;34(11): 3702–9.
71. Kislinger T, Fu C, Huber B, et al. N(epsilon)-(carboxymethyl)lysine adducts of proteins are ligands for receptor for advanced glycation end products that activate cell signaling pathways and modulate gene expression. J Biol Chem 1999; 274(44):31740–9.
72. Kislinger T, Tanji N, Wendt T, et al. Receptor for advanced glycation end products mediates inflammation and enhanced expression of tissue factor in vasculature of diabetic apolipoprotein E-null mice. Arterioscler Thromb Vasc Biol 2001;21(6):905–10.
73. Thornalley PJ. Cell activation by glycated proteins. AGE receptors, receptor recognition factors and functional classification of AGEs. Cell Mol Biol (Noisy-le-grand) 1998;44(7):1013–23.
74. Xie J, Mendez JD, Mendez-Valenzuela V, et al. Cellular signalling of the receptor for advanced glycation end products (RAGE). Cell Signal 2013;25(11):2185–97.
75. Catalfamo DL, Britten TM, Storch DL, et al. Hyperglycemia induced and intrinsic alterations in type 2 diabetes-derived osteoclast function. Oral Dis 2013;19(3): 303–12.
76. Ding KH, Wang ZZ, Hamrick MW, et al. Disordered osteoclast formation in RAGE-deficient mouse establishes an essential role for RAGE in diabetes related bone loss. Biochem Biophys Res Commun 2006;340(4):1091–7.
77. Miyata T, Kawai R, Taketomi S, et al. Possible involvement of advanced glycation end-products in bone resorption. Nephrol Dial Transplant 1996;11(Suppl 5): 54–7.

78. Alikhani M, Alikhani Z, Boyd C, et al. Advanced glycation end products stimulate osteoblast apoptosis via the MAP kinase and cytosolic apoptotic pathways. Bone 2007;40(2):345–53.

79. Saito M, Fujii K, Mori Y, et al. Role of collagen enzymatic and glycation induced cross-links as a determinant of bone quality in spontaneously diabetic WBN/Kob rats. Osteoporos Int 2006;17(10):1514–23.

80. Furst JR, Bandeira LC, Fan WW, et al. Advanced glycation endproducts and bone material strength in type 2 diabetes. J Clin Endocrinol Metab 2016; 101(6):2502–10.

81. Tang SY, Vashishth D. The relative contributions of non-enzymatic glycation and cortical porosity on the fracture toughness of aging bone. J Biomech 2011; 44(2):330–6.

82. Vashishth D, Gibson GJ, Khoury JI, et al. Influence of nonenzymatic glycation on biomechanical properties of cortical bone. Bone 2001;28(2):195–201.

83. Bedi A, Fox AJ, Harris PE, et al. Diabetes mellitus impairs tendon-bone healing after rotator cuff repair. J Shoulder Elbow Surg 2010;19(7):978–88.

84. Frank C, McDonald D, Wilson J, et al. Rabbit medial collateral ligament scar weakness is associated with decreased collagen pyridinoline crosslink density. J Orthop Res 1995;13(2):157–65.

85. St-Pierre J, Buckingham JA, Roebuck SJ, et al. Topology of superoxide production from different sites in the mitochondrial electron transport chain. J Biol Chem 2002;277(47):44784–90.

86. Moussa SA. Oxidative stress in diabetes mellitus. Rom J Biophys 2008;18(3): 225–36.

87. Brand MD. The sites and topology of mitochondrial superoxide production. Exp Gerontol 2010;45(7–8):466–72.

88. Mohazzab KM, Kaminski PM, Wolin MS. NADH oxidoreductase is a major source of superoxide anion in bovine coronary artery endothelium. Am J Physiol 1994;266(6 Pt 2):H2568–72.

89. Morikawa D, Nojiri H, Saita Y, et al. Cytoplasmic reactive oxygen species and SOD1 regulate bone mass during mechanical unloading. J Bone Miner Res 2013;28(11):2368–80.

90. Oikawa A, Siragusa M, Quaini F, et al. Diabetes mellitus induces bone marrow microangiopathy. Arterioscler Thromb Vasc Biol 2010;30(3):498–508.

91. Ha H, Kwak HB, Lee SW, et al. Reactive oxygen species mediate RANK signaling in osteoclasts. Exp Cell Res 2004;301(2):119–27.

92. Yao D, Brownlee M. Hyperglycemia-induced reactive oxygen species increase expression of the receptor for advanced glycation end products (RAGE) and RAGE ligands. Diabetes 2010;59(1):249–55.

93. Almeida M, O'Brien CA. Basic biology of skeletal aging: role of stress response pathways. J Gerontol A Biol Sci Med Sci 2013;68(10):1197–208.

94. Barrow RE, Dasu MR, Ferrando AA, et al. Gene expression patterns in skeletal muscle of thermally injured children treated with oxandrolone. Ann Surg 2003; 237(3):422–8.

95. Yu WK, Li WQ, Li N, et al. Influence of acute hyperglycemia in human sepsis on inflammatory cytokine and counterregulatory hormone concentrations. World J Gastroenterol 2003;9(8):1824–7.

96. Beishuizen A, Thijs LG. The immunoneuroendocrine axis in critical illness: beneficial adaptation or neuroendocrine exhaustion? Curr Opin Crit Care 2004;10(6): 461–7.

97. Bochicchio GV, Salzano L, Joshi M, et al. Admission preoperative glucose is predictive of morbidity and mortality in trauma patients who require immediate operative intervention. Am Surg 2005;71(2):171–4.

98. Dungan KM, Braithwaite SS, Preiser JC. Stress hyperglycaemia. Lancet 2009; 373(9677):1798–807.

99. Marik PE, Bellomo R. Stress hyperglycemia: an essential survival response! Crit Care 2013;17(2):305.

100. Duning T, van den Heuvel I, Dickmann A, et al. Hypoglycemia aggravates critical illness-induced neurocognitive dysfunction. Diabetes Care 2010;33(3): 639–44.

101. Malfitano C, Alba Loureiro TC, Rodrigues B, et al. Hyperglycaemia protects the heart after myocardial infarction: aspects of programmed cell survival and cell death. Eur J Heart Fail 2010;12(7):659–67.

102. Meszaros K, Lang CH, Bagby GJ, et al. In vivo glucose utilization by individual tissues during nonlethal hypermetabolic sepsis. FASEB J 1988;2(15):3083–6.

103. Richards JE, Hutchinson J, Mukherjee K, et al. Stress hyperglycemia and surgical site infection in stable nondiabetic adults with orthopedic injuries. J Trauma Acute Care Surg 2014;76(4):1070–5.

104. Richards JE, Kauffmann RM, Zuckerman SL, et al. Relationship of hyperglycemia and surgical-site infection in orthopaedic surgery. J Bone Joint Surg Am 2012;94(13):1181–6.

105. Karunakar MA, Staples KS. Does stress-induced hyperglycemia increase the risk of perioperative infectious complications in orthopaedic trauma patients? J Orthop Trauma 2010;24(12):752–6.

106. Rau CS, Wu SC, Chen YC, et al. Stress-induced hyperglycemia in diabetes: a cross-sectional analysis to explore the definition based on the trauma registry data. Int J Environ Res Public Health 2017;14(12) [pii:E1527].

107. Rau CS, Wu SC, Chen YC, et al. Higher mortality in trauma patients is associated with stress-induced hyperglycemia, but not diabetic hyperglycemia: a cross-sectional analysis based on a propensity-score matching approach. Int J Environ Res Public Health 2017;14(10) [pii:E1161].

108. American College of Surgeons. Advanced trauma life support. 10th edition. Chicago: American College of Surgeons; 2018.

109. Stamler J, Vaccaro O, Neaton JD, et al. Diabetes, other risk factors, and 12-yr cardiovascular mortality for men screened in the Multiple Risk Factor Intervention Trial. Diabetes Care 1993;16(2):434–44.

110. Rabbitts JA, Nuttall GA, Brown MJ, et al. Cardiac risk of noncardiac surgery after percutaneous coronary intervention with drug-eluting stents. Anesthesiology 2008;109(4):596–604.

111. Rockman CB, Saltzberg SS, Maldonado TS, et al. The safety of carotid endarterectomy in diabetic patients: clinical predictors of adverse outcome. J Vasc Surg 2005;42(5):878–83.

112. Goldman L, Caldera DL, Southwick FS, et al. Cardiac risk factors and complications in non-cardiac surgery. Medicine (Baltimore) 1978;57(4):357–70.

113. Pop-Busui R. What do we know and we do not know about cardiovascular autonomic neuropathy in diabetes. J Cardiovasc Transl Res 2012;5(4):463–78.

114. Tang ZH, Zeng F, Li Z, et al. Association and predictive value analysis for resting heart rate and diabetes mellitus on cardiovascular autonomic neuropathy in general population. J Diabetes Res 2014;2014:215473.

115. Burgos LG, Ebert TJ, Asiddao C, et al. Increased intraoperative cardiovascular morbidity in diabetics with autonomic neuropathy. Anesthesiology 1989;70(4): 591–7.

116. Sivieri R, Veglio M, Chinaglia A, et al. Prevalence of QT prolongation in a type 1 diabetic population and its association with autonomic neuropathy. The Neuropathy Study Group of the Italian Society for the Study of Diabetes. Diabet Med 1993;10(10):920–4.

117. Pop-Busui R. Cardiac autonomic neuropathy in diabetes: a clinical perspective. Diabetes Care 2010;33(2):434–41.

118. Kannel WB, Abbott RD. Incidence and prognosis of unrecognized myocardial infarction. An update on the Framingham study. N Engl J Med 1984;311(18): 1144–7.

119. Wackers FJ, Young LH, Inzucchi SE, et al. Detection of silent myocardial ischemia in asymptomatic diabetic subjects: the DIAD study. Diabetes Care 2004;27(8):1954–61.

120. Juul AB, Wetterslev J, Kofoed-Enevoldsen A. Long-term postoperative mortality in diabetic patients undergoing major non-cardiac surgery. Eur J Anaesthesiol 2004;21(7):523–9.

121. Krolikowska M, Kataja M, Poyhia R, et al. Mortality in diabetic patients undergoing non-cardiac surgery: a 7-year follow-up study. Acta Anaesthesiol Scand 2009;53(6):749–58.

122. Centers for Disease Control and Prevention. Chronic Kidney Disease Surveillance System—United States. Available at: http://www.cdc.gov/ckd.

123. Morduchowicz G, Winkler J, Derazne E, et al. Causes of death in patients with end-stage renal disease treated by dialysis in a center in Israel. Isr J Med Sci 1992;28(11):776–9.

124. Perneger TV, Klag MJ, Whelton PK. Cause of death in patients with end-stage renal disease: death certificates vs registry reports. Am J Public Health 1993; 83(12):1735–8.

125. Tong J, Liu M, Li H, et al. Mortality and associated risk factors in dialysis patients with cardiovascular disease. Kidney Blood Press Res 2016;41(4):479–87.

126. Pinson CW, Schuman ES, Gross GF, et al. Surgery in long-term dialysis patients. Experience with more than 300 cases. Am J Surg 1986;151(5):567–71.

127. Schreiber S, Korzets A, Powsner E, et al. Surgery in chronic dialysis patients. Isr J Med Sci 1995;31(8):479–83.

128. Ozrazgat-Baslanti T, Thottakkara P, Huber M, et al. Acute and chronic kidney disease and cardiovascular mortality after major surgery. Ann Surg 2016; 264(6):987–96.

129. Galbusera M, Remuzzi G, Boccardo P. Treatment of bleeding in dialysis patients. Semin Dial 2009;22(3):279–86.

130. Holden RM, Harman GJ, Wang M, et al. Major bleeding in hemodialysis patients. Clin J Am Soc Nephrol 2008;3(1):105–10.

131. Hovaguimian F, Myles PS. Restrictive versus liberal transfusion strategy in the perioperative and acute care settings: a context-specific systematic review and meta-analysis of randomized controlled trials. Anesthesiology 2016; 125(1):46–61.

132. Beks PJ, Mackaay AJ, de Neeling JN, et al. Peripheral arterial disease in relation to glycaemic level in an elderly Caucasian population: the Hoorn study. Diabetologia 1995;38(1):86–96.

133. Elhadd TA, Robb R, Jung RT, et al. Pilot study of prevalence of asymptomatic peripheral arterial occlusive disease in patients with diabetes attending a hospital clinic. Pract Diabetes Int 1999;16:163–6.

134. Selvin E, Marinopoulos S, Berkenblit G, et al. Meta-analysis: glycosylated hemoglobin and cardiovascular disease in diabetes mellitus. Ann Intern Med 2004; 141(6):421–31.

135. Prompers L, Huijberts M, Apelqvist J, et al. High prevalence of ischaemia, infection and serious comorbidity in patients with diabetic foot disease in Europe. Baseline results from the Eurodiale study. Diabetologia 2007;50(1):18–25.

136. Wukich DK, Shen W, Raspovic KM, et al. Noninvasive arterial testing in patients with diabetes: a guide for foot and ankle surgeons. Foot Ankle Int 2015;36(12): 1391–9.

137. Imagama S, Matsuyama Y, Sakai Y, et al. An arterial pulse examination is not sufficient for diagnosis of peripheral arterial disease in lumbar spinal canal stenosis: a prospective multicenter study. Spine (Phila Pa 1976) 2011;36(15): 1204–10.

138. Wukich DK, Joseph A, Ryan M, et al. Outcomes of ankle fractures in patients with uncomplicated versus complicated diabetes. Foot Ankle Int 2011;32(2): 120–30.

139. Jeffcoate WJ, Rasmussen LM, Hofbauer LC, et al. Medial arterial calcification in diabetes and its relationship to neuropathy. Diabetologia 2009;52(12):2478–88.

140. Albers JW, Pop-Busui R. Diabetic neuropathy: mechanisms, emerging treatments, and subtypes. Curr Neurol Neurosci Rep 2014;14(8):473.

141. Dyck PJ, Albers JW, Andersen H, et al. Diabetic polyneuropathies: update on research definition, diagnostic criteria and estimation of severity. Diabetes Metab Res Rev 2011;27(7):620–8.

142. Malik RA, Veves A, Tesfaye S, et al. Small fibre neuropathy: role in the diagnosis of diabetic sensorimotor polyneuropathy. Diabetes Metab Res Rev 2011;27(7): 678–84.

143. Young MJ, Boulton AJ, MacLeod AF, et al. A multicentre study of the prevalence of diabetic peripheral neuropathy in the United Kingdom hospital clinic population. Diabetologia 1993;36(2):150–4.

144. Suder NC, Wukich DK. Prevalence of diabetic neuropathy in patients undergoing foot and ankle surgery. Foot Ankle Spec 2012;5(2):97–101.

145. Feldman EL, Stevens MJ, Thomas PK, et al. A practical two-step quantitative clinical and electrophysiological assessment for the diagnosis and staging of diabetic neuropathy. Diabetes Care 1994;17(11):1281–9.

146. Game FL, Catlow R, Jones GR, et al. Audit of acute Charcot's disease in the UK: the CDUK study. Diabetologia 2012;55(1):32–5.

147. Rajbhandari SM, Jenkins RC, Davies C, et al. Charcot neuroarthropathy in diabetes mellitus. Diabetologia 2002;45(8):1085–96.

148. Jeffcoate WJ. Charcot neuro-osteoarthropathy. Diabetes Metab Res Rev 2008; 24(Suppl 1):S62–5.

149. Sanders LJ, Frykberg RG. Charcot foot. In: O'Neal LW, Bowker JH, editors. The diabetic foot. 5th edition. St Louis (MO): Mosby Year Books; 1993. p. 149–80.

150. Young MJ, Marshall A, Adams JE, et al. Osteopenia, neurological dysfunction, and the development of Charcot neuroarthropathy. Diabetes Care 1995;18(1): 34–8.

151. Rix M, Andreassen H, Eskildsen P. Impact of peripheral neuropathy on bone density in patients with type 1 diabetes. Diabetes Care 1999;22(5):827–31.

152. Elefteriou F, Ahn JD, Takeda S, et al. Leptin regulation of bone resorption by the sympathetic nervous system and CART. Nature 2005;434(7032):514–20.
153. Takeda S, Elefteriou F, Levasseur R, et al. Leptin regulates bone formation via the sympathetic nervous system. Cell 2002;111(3):305–17.
154. Kruger L, Silverman JD, Mantyh PW, et al. Peripheral patterns of calcitonin-gene-related peptide general somatic sensory innervation: cutaneous and deep terminations. J Comp Neurol 1989;280(2):291–302.
155. Schinke T, Liese S, Priemel M, et al. Decreased bone formation and osteopenia in mice lacking alpha-calcitonin gene-related peptide. J Bone Miner Res 2004; 19(12):2049–56.
156. Gough A, Abraha H, Li F, et al. Measurement of markers of osteoclast and osteoblast activity in patients with acute and chronic diabetic Charcot neuroarthropathy. Diabet Med 1997;14(7):527–31.
157. La Fontaine J, Harkless LB, Sylvia VL, et al. Levels of endothelial nitric oxide synthase and calcitonin gene-related peptide in the Charcot foot: a pilot study. J Foot Ankle Surg 2008;47(5):424–9.
158. Christensen TM, Bulow J, Simonsen L, et al. Bone mineral density in diabetes mellitus patients with and without a Charcot foot. Clin Physiol Funct Imaging 2010;30(2):130–4.
159. Greenhagen RM, Wukich DK, Jung RH, et al. Peripheral and central bone mineral density in Charcot's neuroarthropathy compared in diabetic and nondiabetic populations. J Am Podiatr Med Assoc 2012;102(3):213–22.
160. Wukich DK, Crim BE, Frykberg RG, et al. Neuropathy and poorly controlled diabetes increase the rate of surgical site infection after foot and ankle surgery. J Bone Joint Surg Am 2014;96(10):832–9.
161. Wukich DK, Lowery NJ, McMillen RL, et al. Postoperative infection rates in foot and ankle surgery: a comparison of patients with and without diabetes mellitus. J Bone Joint Surg Am 2010;92(2):287–95.
162. Wukich DK, McMillen RL, Lowery NJ, et al. Surgical site infections after foot and ankle surgery: a comparison of patients with and without diabetes. Diabetes Care 2011;34(10):2211–3.
163. Parkhouse N, Le Quesne PM. Impaired neurogenic vascular response in patients with diabetes and neuropathic foot lesions. N Engl J Med 1988;318(20): 1306–9.
164. da Silva L, Carvalho E, Cruz MT. Role of neuropeptides in skin inflammation and its involvement in diabetic wound healing. Expert Opin Biol Ther 2010;10(10): 1427–39.
165. Ekstrand AJ, Cao R, Bjorndahl M, et al. Deletion of neuropeptide Y (NPY) 2 receptor in mice results in blockage of NPY-induced angiogenesis and delayed wound healing. Proc Natl Acad Sci U S A 2003;100(10):6033–8.
166. Toda M, Suzuki T, Hosono K, et al. Roles of calcitonin gene-related peptide in facilitation of wound healing and angiogenesis. Biomed Pharmacother 2008; 62(6):352–9.
167. Holick MF, Binkley NC, Bischoff-Ferrari HA, et al. Evaluation, treatment, and prevention of vitamin D deficiency: an Endocrine Society clinical practice guideline. J Clin Endocrinol Metab 2011;96(7):1911–30.
168. Forrest KY, Stuhldreher WL. Prevalence and correlates of vitamin D deficiency in US adults. Nutr Res 2011;31(1):48–54.
169. Maier GS, Jakob P, Horas K, et al. Vitamin D deficiency in orthopaedic patients: a single center analysis. Acta Orthop Belg 2013;79(5):587–91.

170. Hood MA, Murtha YM, Della Rocca GJ, et al. Prevalence of low vitamin D levels in patients with orthopedic trauma. Am J Orthop (Belle Mead NJ) 2016;45(7): E522–6.

171. Yoho RM, Frerichs J, Dodson NB, et al. A comparison of vitamin D levels in nondiabetic and diabetic patient populations. J Am Podiatr Med Assoc 2009; 99(1):35–41.

172. Brinker MR, O'Connor DP. Outcomes of tibial nonunion in older adults following treatment using the Ilizarov method. J Orthop Trauma 2007;21(9):634–42.

173. LeBoff MS, Hawkes WG, Glowacki J, et al. Vitamin D-deficiency and post-fracture changes in lower extremity function and falls in women with hip fractures. Osteoporos Int 2008;19(9):1283–90.

174. Bischoff-Ferrari HA, Dawson-Hughes B, Willett WC, et al. Effect of Vitamin D on falls: a meta-analysis. JAMA 2004;291(16):1999–2006.

175. Robertson DS, Jenkins T, Murtha YM, et al. Effectiveness of vitamin D therapy in orthopaedic trauma patients. J Orthop Trauma 2015;29(11):e451–3.

176. Doenst T, Wijeysundera D, Karkouti K, et al. Hyperglycemia during cardiopulmonary bypass is an independent risk factor for mortality in patients undergoing cardiac surgery. J Thorac Cardiovasc Surg 2005;130(4):1144.

177. Kwon S, Thompson R, Dellinger P, et al. Importance of perioperative glycemic control in general surgery: a report from the Surgical Care and Outcomes Assessment Program. Ann Surg 2013;257(1):8–14.

178. Mraovic B, Suh D, Jacovides C, et al. Perioperative hyperglycemia and postoperative infection after lower limb arthroplasty. J Diabetes Sci Technol 2011;5(2): 412–8.

179. Ouattara A, Lecomte P, Le Manach Y, et al. Poor intraoperative blood glucose control is associated with a worsened hospital outcome after cardiac surgery in diabetic patients. Anesthesiology 2005;103(4):687–94.

180. Delamaire M, Maugendre D, Moreno M, et al. Impaired leucocyte functions in diabetic patients. Diabet Med 1997;14(1):29–34.

181. Marhoffer W, Stein M, Maeser E, et al. Impairment of polymorphonuclear leukocyte function and metabolic control of diabetes. Diabetes Care 1992;15(2): 256–60.

182. Richards JE, Kauffmann RM, Obremskey WT, et al. Stress-induced hyperglycemia as a risk factor for surgical-site infection in nondiabetic orthopedic trauma patients admitted to the intensive care unit. J Orthop Trauma 2013;27(1):16–21.

183. Sadoskas D, Suder NC, Wukich DK. Perioperative glycemic control and the effect on surgical site infections in diabetic patients undergoing foot and ankle surgery. Foot Ankle Spec 2016;9(1):24–30.

184. Standards of medical care for patients with diabetes mellitus. Diabetes Care 1989;12(5):365–8.

185. Cakmak M, Cakmak N, Cetemen S, et al. The value of admission glycosylated hemoglobin level in patients with acute myocardial infarction. Can J Cardiol 2008;24(5):375–8.

186. Domek N, Dux K, Pinzur M, et al. Association between hemoglobin A1c and surgical morbidity in elective foot and ankle surgery. J Foot Ankle Surg 2016;55(5): 939–43.

187. Dronge AS, Perkal MF, Kancir S, et al. Long-term glycemic control and postoperative infectious complications. Arch Surg 2006;141(4):375–80 [discussion: 380].

188. Halkos ME, Puskas JD, Lattouf OM, et al. Elevated preoperative hemoglobin A1c level is predictive of adverse events after coronary artery bypass surgery. J Thorac Cardiovasc Surg 2008;136(3):631–40.

189. Han HS, Kang SB. Relations between long-term glycemic control and postoperative wound and infectious complications after total knee arthroplasty in type 2 diabetics. Clin Orthop Surg 2013;5(2):118–23.

190. Hwang JS, Kim SJ, Bamne AB, et al. Do glycemic markers predict occurrence of complications after total knee arthroplasty in patients with diabetes? Clin Orthop Relat Res 2015;473(5):1726–31.

191. Jupiter DC, Humphers JM, Shibuya N. Trends in postoperative infection rates and their relationship to glycosylated hemoglobin levels in diabetic patients undergoing foot and ankle surgery. J Foot Ankle Surg 2014;53(3):307–11.

192. O'Sullivan CJ, Hynes N, Mahendran B, et al. Haemoglobin A1c (HbA1C) in non-diabetic and diabetic vascular patients. Is HbA1C an independent risk factor and predictor of adverse outcome? Eur J Vasc Endovasc Surg 2006;32(2): 188–97.

193. Yang MH, Jaeger M, Baxter M, et al. Postoperative dysglycemia in elective non-diabetic surgical patients: a prospective observational study. Can J Anaesth 2016;63(12):1319–34.

194. Association American Diabetes. Updates to the standards of medical care in diabetes-2018. Diabetes Care 2018;41(9):2045–7.

195. Shibuya N, Humphers JM, Fluhman BL, et al. Factors associated with nonunion, delayed union, and malunion in foot and ankle surgery in diabetic patients. J Foot Ankle Surg 2013;52(2):207–11.

196. Trussell J, Gerkin R, Coates B, et al. Impact of a patient care pathway protocol on surgical site infection rates in cardiothoracic surgery patients. Am J Surg 2008;196(6):883–9 [discussion: 889].

197. Umpierrez GE, Smiley D, Jacobs S, et al. Randomized study of basal-bolus insulin therapy in the inpatient management of patients with type 2 diabetes undergoing general surgery (RABBIT 2 surgery). Diabetes Care 2011;34(2): 256–61.

198. Agos F, Shoda C, Bransford D. Part II: managing perioperative hyperglycemia in total hip and knee replacement surgeries. Nurs Clin North Am 2014;49(3): 299–308.

199. van den Berghe G, Wouters P, Weekers F, et al. Intensive insulin therapy in critically ill patients. N Engl J Med 2001;345(19):1359–67.

200. NICE-SUGAR Study Investigators, Finfer S, Chittock DR, Su SY. Intensive versus conventional glucose control in critically ill patients. N Engl J Med 2009;360: 1283–97.

201. Sudhakaran S, Surani SR. Guidelines for perioperative management of the diabetic patient. Surg Res Pract 2015;2015:284063.

202. American Diabetes Association. Standards of medical care in diabetes–2009. Diabetes Care 2009;32(Suppl 1):S13–61.

203. Golightly LK, Jones MA, Hamamura DH, et al. Management of diabetes mellitus in hospitalized patients: efficiency and effectiveness of sliding-scale insulin therapy. Pharmacotherapy 2006;26(10):1421–32.

204. Hirsch IB. Sliding scale insulin–time to stop sliding. JAMA 2009;301(2):213–4.

205. Queale WS, Seidler AJ, Brancati FL. Glycemic control and sliding scale insulin use in medical inpatients with diabetes mellitus. Arch Intern Med 1997;157(5): 545–52.

206. Wexler DJ, Meigs JB, Cagliero E, et al. Prevalence of hyper- and hypoglycemia among inpatients with diabetes: a national survey of 44 U.S. hospitals. Diabetes Care 2007;30(2):367–9.
207. Moghissi ES. Addressing hyperglycemia from hospital admission to discharge. Curr Med Res Opin 2010;26(3):589–98.
208. Mraovic B, Hipszer BR, Epstein RH, et al. Preadmission hyperglycemia is an independent risk factor for in-hospital symptomatic pulmonary embolism after major orthopedic surgery. J Arthroplasty 2010;25(1):64–70.
209. Machino M, Yukawa Y, Ito K, et al. Risk factors for poor outcome of cervical laminoplasty for cervical spondylotic myelopathy in patients with diabetes. J Bone Joint Surg Am 2014;96(24):2049–55.
210. Chrastil J, Anderson MB, Stevens V, et al. Is hemoglobin A1c or perioperative hyperglycemia predictive of periprosthetic joint infection or death following primary total joint arthroplasty? J Arthroplasty 2015;30(7):1197–202.
211. SooHoo NF, Krenek L, Eagan MJ, et al. Complication rates following open reduction and internal fixation of ankle fractures. J Bone Joint Surg Am 2009;91(5):1042–9.
212. Gortler H, Rusyn J, Godbout C, et al. Diabetes and healing outcomes in lower extremity fractures: a systematic review. Injury 2018;49(2):177–83.
213. Aderinto J, Keating JF. Intramedullary nailing of fractures of the tibia in diabetics. J Bone Joint Surg Br 2008;90(5):638–42.
214. Kline AJ, Gruen GS, Pape HC, et al. Early complications following the operative treatment of pilon fractures with and without diabetes. Foot Ankle Int 2009;30(11):1042–7.
215. Blotter RH, Connolly E, Wasan A, et al. Acute complications in the operative treatment of isolated ankle fractures in patients with diabetes mellitus. Foot Ankle Int 1999;20(11):687–94.
216. Flynn JM, Rodriguez-del Rio F, Piza PA. Closed ankle fractures in the diabetic patient. Foot Ankle Int 2000;21(4):311–9.
217. Jones KB, Maiers-Yelden KA, Marsh JL, et al. Ankle fractures in patients with diabetes mellitus. J Bone Joint Surg Br 2005;87(4):489–95.
218. Guo JJ, Yang H, Xu Y, et al. Results after immediate operations of closed ankle fractures in patients with preoperatively neglected type 2 diabetes. Injury 2009;40(8):894–6.

Atypical Wounds; Hyperbaric Oxygen Therapy

Carol Deane Benedict Mitnick, MD[a], Kelly Johnson-Arbor, MD, FUHM[b],*

KEYWORDS

- Hyperbaric oxygenation • Wound healing • Diabetes • Peripheral vascular disease
- Atypical ulcers • Vasculitis • Coagulopathy • Autoimmune disorders

KEY POINTS

- Chronic ulcers that have not responded to appropriate wound care should be considered for some of the less common etiologies of ulcers.
- Proper identification of etiology of legs ulcers is important for appropriate management and treatment of patients.
- Delayed progression of wound healing in chronic wounds can be secondary to their inability to transition from the inflammatory phase to the proliferation phase.
- Hyperbaric oxygen therapy involves the systemic administration of oxygen at pressures greater than sea level.
- Hyperbaric oxygen therapy is an adjunctive treatment of selected diabetic foot ulcerations that have failed to respond to standard conservative treatments.

In the United States in 2015, an estimated 30.3 million people (9.4% of the US population) had diabetes and another 84.1 million adults aged 18 years or older had prediabetes (33.9% of the adult US population).[1] With this large diabetic population, it stands to reason that patients with other diseases are more likely to also have comorbid disease with diabetes. Therefore, diabetic patients presenting with lower extremity ulcers also should be considered for other diagnoses that may be contributing to, or be the actual cause of their lower extremity ulcers. For example, patients with diabetes with comorbid rheumatoid arthritis are more likely than those without rheumatoid arthritis to have lower extremity ulcers.[2]

The most common etiology of leg ulcers is of venous origin, followed by arterial occlusive disease and neuropathic (diabetic) ulcers.[3,4] Chronic ulcers (defined as

Disclosures: The authors have nothing to disclose.
[a] Division of Rheumatology, Immunology and Allergy, Center for Wound Healing, MedStar Georgetown University Hospital, 3800 Reservoir Road Northwest, 3PHC, Suite 3004, Washington, DC 20007, USA; [b] MedStar Georgetown University Hospital, 3800 Reservoir Road Northwest, Washington, DC 20007, USA
* Corresponding author.
E-mail address: kkja@me.com

ulcers present for more than 4 weeks[3]) that are nonresponsive to 3 months of appropriate wound care should be considered for some of the less common etiologies of ulcers.[4,5] A multicenter prospective study of consecutive patients presenting with lower extremity ulcers found the mean age of patients with uncommon ulcers was 65.6 years and the mean duration of their ulcer was 5.5 years.[4] In a study of patient's who presented to a tertiary wound center, it has been reported that the incidence of ulcers with atypical origin ranges from 2.1% to as high as 23% of patients found to have an associated immune disease.[4,6,7] Proper identification of the etiology of legs ulcers is important for appropriate management and treatment of patients. Incorrect treatment may cause significant harm[3] with these wounds having a significant impact on mortality,[5,8] as well as causing pain, and affecting patient-reported psychosocial well-being and quality of life.[5,9]

Wound healing is strictly regulated by multiple growth factors and cytokines released at the wound site[10] and consists of 3 phases: (1) hemostasis and inflammation, (2) proliferation, and (3) maturation and remodeling.[11] Although acute wounds follow these phases, chronic wounds do not progress through this orderly process having lost the ideal synchrony of events which prevents normal wound healing.[10] One reason for delayed progression of wound healing in chronic wounds is their inability to transition from the inflammatory phase to the proliferation phase.[5,7] Some of the diseases that are believed to contribute to the arrest in the inflammatory phase of these atypical ulcers includes, but not limited to vasculitis, pyoderma gangrenosum (PG), calciphylaxis, and systemic autoimmune/connective tissue disorders.[5-7,10]

Ulcers due to vasculitis can be secondary to multiple underlying etiologies including drugs; autoimmune disorders such as systemic lupus erythematous, antineutrophil cytoplasmic antibody–associated vasculitis, rheumatoid arthritis, and thromboangiitis obliterans (previously known as Buerger disease); and infections such as hepatitis C leading to mixed cryoglobulinemia and hepatitis B associated with polyarteritis nodosa.[3,5,6,12]

Atypical ulcers secondary to a coagulopathy include autoimmune diseases, such as antiphospholipid syndrome in which there is occlusion of the small dermal vessels, as well as those secondary to genetic prothrombotic states including prothrombin gene mutation, factor V Leiden mutation, plasminogen activator inhibitor, and MTHFR gene mutation.[3-5] Hematological disorders, such as sickle cell anemia, thrombotic thrombocytopenic purpura, and essential thrombocythemia, also are known to cause lower extremity ulcers with microvascular thrombosis the most likely pathogenetic factor.[3]

In patients with underlying connective tissue disorders, the pathophysiology of the atypical ulcer may be both coagulopathy and inflammatory (vasculitis) and the combination of these 2 conditions predisposes for necrosis. Both the use of antiplatelet and/or anticoagulation and immunosuppressive agents may be needed in treatment of these ulcers.[3,5,12,13]

Pyoderma gangrenosum (PG), a neutrophilic dermatosis resulting in cutaneous ulcerations,[14] is another important diagnosis to consider in the nonhealing wound. At this time the diagnosis of pyoderma is one of exclusion and there currently are no uniformly accepted diagnostic criteria for PG.[15,16] However, there are 2 sets of proposed criteria for diagnosis of PG. Su and colleagues[15] proposed criteria that require both 2 major criteria and at least 2 minor criteria be met (**Box 1**). This diagnostic criterion maintains ulcerative PG as a diagnosis of exclusion. More recently a Delphi consensus of international experts proposed a diagnostic criterion to address the concern that diagnosis of exclusion is not compatible with clinical decision making or for inclusion for clinical trials. This proposed diagnostic criterion includes 1 major criterion and 4 of 8 minor criteria be met for a diagnosis of ulcerative PG.[16]

> **Box 1**
> **Proposed criteria for the diagnosis of pyoderma gangrenosum**
>
> *Major criteria*
>
> 1. Rapid progression of a painful, necrolytic, cutaneous ulcer with an irregular, violaceous, undermined border
>
> 2. Other causes of cutaneous ulceration have been ruled out.
>
> *Minor criteria*
>
> 1. History suggestive of pathergy or clinical findings of cribriform scarring
>
> 2. Systemic diseases associated with PG
>
> 3. Histopathologic findings (sterile dermal neutrophilia ± mixed inflammation ± lymphocytic vasculitis)
>
> 4. Treatment response to systemic steroids
>
> *Adapted from* Su WPD, Davis MDP, Weenig RH, et al. Pyoderma gangrenosum: clinicopathologic correlation and proposed diagnostic criteria. Int J Dermatol 2004 Nov;43(11):791; with permission.

To help determine the etiology of chronic ulcers, evaluation of patients should include a thorough history and physical examination, screening laboratory tests, and biopsy.[6] If biopsy of the ulcer is intended to determine an uncommon etiology, the biopsy should be performed at the ulcer edge and should include epidermis to establish diagnosis and rule out malignancy. One specimen should be sent for direct immunofluorescence testing and another specimen sent for hematoxylin & eosin staining with the border of the ulcer as the equator of the biopsy. Deep tissue culture also should be sent and tested for acid-fast bacilli, fungi, and bacteria. The location of the ulcer is one factor to be included when considering ulcers etiology. According to Labropoulou and colleagues, most atypical ulcers were located in the medial lower calf.[4] Venous leg ulcers predominantly occur above the malleoli, with arterial ulcers occurring often at the toes, shin, and over pressure points. Diabetic ulcers often occur over pressure points, especially the distal metatarsal joints.[3,17] An irregular border, black necrosis, erythema, or bluish or purplish discoloration of adjacent skin may be suggestive of vasculitis.[3]

A patient's history of repeated thrombophlebitis or unexplained thrombosis at young age may suggest a hypercoagulable state and is an indication for screening for clotting disorders.[3] Screening laboratory tests to investigate for vasculitis and/or autoimmune etiology include antinuclear antibody, rheumatoid factor, anticyclic citrullinated peptide, antineutrophil cytoplasmic antibodies, and hepatitis B and hepatitis C. Screening laboratory tests for prothrombotic states include anticardiolipin antibodies, anti–β_2-glycoprotein I antibody, lupus anticoagulant, prothrombin gene mutation, factor V Leiden mutation, antithrombin III, and protein C and protein S.[3,5]

In patients with findings consistent with atypical ulcer, referral to a multidisciplinary wound healing center is appropriate and is globally considered the standard of care for treatment of complex wounds. This multidisciplinary approach allows providers of different backgrounds, knowledge, and experience to work together to ensure that patients with a complex wound receive medical, nutritional, surgical, and biomechanical evaluation and treatment. This approach has led to improved clinical outcomes, including a decrease in major amputations.[18,19]

In summary, diabetic patients who present with chronic ulcers that continue to be nonhealing despite appropriate wound care should be evaluated for less common etiologies of the ulcer as well as comorbid disease that may be hindering and/or contributing to the ulcer to ensure proper diagnosis and treatment of these patients.

Hyperbaric oxygen therapy (HBO) is a treatment in which patients breathe 100% oxygen while pressurized to a depth greater than sea level. The use of hyperbaric pressurization as a treatment of medical conditions dates back to the 1600s, prior to the discovery of oxygen.[20] Currently, HBO is used as a primary treatment of decompression sickness, air embolism, and carbon monoxide poisoning. It also is used as an adjunctive treatment of additional medical conditions, including compromised grafts and flaps, chronic refractory osteomyelitis, and diabetic foot ulcerations (DFUs). The Undersea and Hyperbaric Medical Society (UHMS) currently recommends the use of HBO as a treatment of the following conditions[21]:

1. Air or gas embolism
2. Decompression sickness
3. Acute carbon monoxide poisoning
4. Arterial insufficiencies, including enhancement of healing in selected problem wounds
5. Radiation-induced soft tissue and bone necrosis
6. Intracranial abscess
7. Clostridial myonecrosis
8. Necrotizing soft tissue infections
9. Compromised grafts and flaps
10. Crush injuries and compartment syndromes
11. Chronic refractory osteomyelitis
12. Thermal burns
13. Severe anemia where transfusion is impossible due to religious or medical concerns
14. Idiopathic sudden sensorineural hearing loss

Because peripheral arterial disease is a major contributing factor in more than 50% of lower extremity diabetic wounds, HBO is often used as a treatment of DFUs with the associated microvascular arterial insufficiency. There are multiple mechanisms of action of HBO in the treatment of DFUs. The administration of oxygen under pressure leads to greatly increased systemic oxygen concentrations; during treatment, the Pao_2 can exceed 2000 mm Hg, and tissue oxygen concentrations can range from 200 mm Hg to 400 mm Hg.[22] Systemic hyperoxygenation stimulates the generation of reactive oxygen and reactive nitrogen species, which in turn leads to increased wound growth factor synthesis and stem cell mobilization as well as collagen deposition and fibroblast proliferation. Production of vascular endothelial growth factor, the most specific known growth factor related to neovascularization, increases by 40% under hyperbaric conditions.[23] The end result of this process is neovascularization; in patients with DFUs due to underlying peripheral vascular disease, the administration of HBO may lead to improved vascular density in the affected wound tissue. Hyperbaric-mediated increases in reactive oxygen and nitrogen species also result in a decrease in the systemic inflammatory response in tissues.[22] Soft tissue penetration of some antibiotics is enhanced under hyperbaric conditions.[24] In addition, the vasoconstrictive properties of HBO can lead to edema reduction and improved tissue viability in acute wounds, such as compromised skin flaps and grafts.

HBO is administered while a patient is enclosed within a hyperbaric chamber. These chambers, composed of steel and acrylic components, commonly are located within outpatient wound centers in the United States and are utilized as an adjunctive wound healing modality. Monoplace hyperbaric chambers can accommodate 1 patient;

multiplace hyperbaric chambers can accommodate multiple patients. In the United States, monoplace chambers are the most commonly encountered hyperbaric treatment vessels in hospital settings. During hyperbaric treatments, patients sit or lay supine in the hyperbaric chamber and breathe 100% oxygen for the duration of the treatment. Hyperbaric treatments generally are scheduled on a daily basis; most hyperbaric chambers in the United States operate during weekday business hours only, but some facilities may offer weekend or after-hours treatments for emergent conditions, such as compromised skin flaps or grafts. Patients generally receive between 40 to 60 hyperbaric treatments over a 2-month to 3-month course, because hyperbaric-induced neovascularization generally does not occur for at least a month after treatments begin.[25] Each hyperbaric treatment is approximately 2 hours in duration; patients typically sleep or watch a movie during the treatment. The HBO treatment course typically is tailored to each individual patient; some patients may end their treatment course earlier than expected based on a more rapid course of healing. Despite the lengthy time commitment and need to present to the hospital for daily treatments, HBO has not been associated with decrements in patient quality of life.[26] The use of traditional medical equipment and implanted devices in the hyperbaric environment poses unique challenges related to the inability of many modern medical devices (including intravenous pumps and ventilators) to withstand the typical pressurization encountered in the hyperbaric chamber. Most monoplace chambers are designed to treat the outpatient population only, because they are unable to accommodate patients who are undergoing treatment with mechanical ventilation or continuous intravenous infusions. Some implanted medical devices are unsuitable for use in the hyperbaric environment, due to fire safety concerns. Fortunately, many pacemaker manufacturers have tested their devices under pressure, and thus permanent pacemakers often are not regarded as a contraindication to hyperbaric compression. Topical oxygen therapy involves administration of oxygen via a bag, boot, or other device to a specific area of the body, most commonly the lower extremity. Advantages of topical oxygen therapy include a lower cost than traditional HBO and ease of use: topical oxygen can be administered in an out-of-hospital setting, such as a private residence or nursing facility.[27] Unlike HBO, topical oxygen therapy is not associated with the potential for systemic oxygen toxicity. Topical oxygen delivery systems, however, generally do not achieve the high pressures found in hyperbaric chamber environments, and at this time there is not sufficient high-quality evidence to support the use of topical oxygen therapy as a medical treatment.[27,28] Because of this, the procedure often is not reimbursed by insurance carriers.

For decades, HBO has been used as a treatment of DFUs that have failed to respond to conventional therapies. HBO is not a primary treatment of DFUs; rather, it should be used as part of a comprehensive, multispecialty treatment wound treatment program. Use of a multidisciplinary treatment program for DFUs can reduce amputation rates by more than 50%.[29] Therefore, it is highly important for wound care physicians and podiatrists to consider and treat other potential complicating factors in patients with DFUs and not to rely on HBO as the solitary treatment of the condition. In the United States, the Centers for Medicare & Medicaid Services (CMS) authorizes the use of HBO for treatment of DFUs only if a patient also has undergone evaluation and treatment with topical wound care, débridement of devitalized tissue, offloading of affected areas, nutritional optimization, glucose optimization, control of any associated infections, and evaluation and attempted correction of any vascular problems in the affected extremity.[30] In addition, CMS requires that diabetic foot wounds are classified as Wagner grade 3 or greater (eg, extending to bone, tendon, or joint with associated osteomyelitis, tendonitis, or joint infection) to qualify for HBO.[31]

In multiple studies, HBO administration has been reported to both facilitate healing and decrease the rate of major amputations in patients with DFUs, through the aforementioned mechanisms of action.[32–35] Using Grading of Recommendations Assessment, Development and Evaluation (GRADE) methodology, the UHMS performed a systematic review of available literature regarding the use of HBO for DFUs and determined that HBO is beneficial in promoting healing and preventing amputation in patients with Wagner grade 3 or greater DFUs who have not shown signs of improvement after 30 days of standard conventional therapy.[36] In patients with Wagner grade 2 ulcers (eg, a deeper ulcer extending to tendon, joint, or bone but without associated infection), there was not sufficient evidence to support the use of HBO as an adjunctive treatment, and the investigators recommended against the use of HBO for this group of patients due to lack of evidence.[36] The investigators suggested further that patients with Wagner grade 3 or greater DFUs who have had recent surgical debridement of the affected area may benefit from postoperative use of HBO in addition to standard treatments to reduce the risk of amputation or impaired healing.

Several recently published studies have questioned the efficacy and effectiveness of HBO for the treatment of diabetic foot wounds. In 2013, Margolis and colleagues[37] compared the effectiveness of HBO with other wound care modalities in the treatment of patients with nonhealing DFUs. Inclusion criteria included patients with Wagner grade 2 or greater diabetic foot wounds. The results of this study indicated that patients who received HBO were more likely to have an amputation and were less likely to heal. In 2016, Fedorko and colleagues[38] studied whether patients with Wagner grade 2 to 4 DFUs would experience a need for major amputation when administered HBO and concluded that HBO did not reduce criteria for amputation. Santema and colleagues[39] studied the use of HBO for wound healing and limb salvage in patients with Wagner grade 2 to 4 DFUs. In this study, HBO did not significantly improve wound healing and limb salvage. Limitations of all 3 studies include the studies' inclusion criteria of patients with Wagner grade 2 DFUs; there is no evidence that patients with Wagner grade 2 DFUs benefit from the use of HBO, and this patient population generally is not treated with HBO in the United States. There were significant numbers of patients with Wagner grade 2 DFUs, however, included in all 3 studies discussed previously. In addition, the criteria for amputation used for determining primary outcome in Fedorko and colleagues'[38] study were based on evaluation of participant data and digital photographs by a vascular surgeon; actual amputation rates were not discussed in the study. Limitations in Santema and colleagues'[39] study included a low rate of treatment completion in the HBO group; despite this, the rate of major amputation was reduced in the group that received the full prescribed course of HBO. This result indicates that HBO may truly result in reduced amputation rates when a full treatment regimen is completed. Based on the results of these studies as well as the UHMS GRADE analysis of HBO for DFUs, it is evident that selected patient populations (those with Wagner grade 3 or greater DFUs) seem to benefit from the use of HBO, but the generalized application of HBO to all patients with Wagner grade 2 DFUs cannot be recommended.

Adverse effects of HBO are rare. Middle ear barotrauma is the most common complication of HBO; this is generally self-limited and can be prevented by carefully instructing patients on appropriate ear pressure equalization techniques. Central nervous system oxygen toxicity may result in seizures; however, seizures rarely are encountered in clinical hyperbaric practice. The risk of central nervous system oxygen toxicity may be reduced by the use of intermittent air breathing periods during each hyperbaric treatment. In diabetic patients, hyperbaric pressurization may result in hypoglycemia. Some patients may experience a temporary myopic shift during their hyperbaric treatment course, and patients with a history of anxiety or claustrophobia may exhibit confinement anxiety during hyperbaric treatments. Finally, because the hyperbaric environment is oxygen enriched by definition, fire safety is of paramount importance. Careful assessment and mitigation of any potential fire risk factors must be performed and maintained during each hyperbaric treatment. Fire-related fatalities have occurred in hyperbaric chambers due to the presence of static electricity, electrical shorts, and tobacco use within the hyperbaric environment.[40] The National Fire Protection Association (NFPA) publishes standards for fire safety in health care facilities; hospital-based hyperbaric chambers must follow these standards. In accordance with NFPA regulations, patients may not wear garments of less than 50% cotton in monoplace hyperbaric chambers; in addition, patients may not bring cell phones, personal entertainment devices, personal warming devices, or any other items that may ignite or fuel a fire.[41]

When administered correctly, HBO is a safe procedure with minimal adverse effects. In patients with Wagner grade 3 or greater DFUs, HBO administration may result in reduced rates of major amputation and impaired wound healing, but these results are not generalizable to patients with less severe DFUs. Additional patient groups, including patients with Wagner grade 3 DFUs who have undergone surgical débridement of the wounds, also may be candidates for HBO. In the DFU patient population, careful patient selection and judicious use of hyperbaric oxygenation can result in optimal patient outcomes when combined with a comprehensive and multidisciplinary approach at limb salvage.

REFERENCES

1. National Diabetes Fact Sheet, 2017. Available at: https://www.cdc.gov/diabetes/pdfs/data/statistics/national-diabetes-statistics-report.pdf. Accessed January 14, 2019.

2. Bartels CM, Saucier JM, Thorpe CT, et al. Monitoring diabetes in patients with and without rheumatoid arthritis: a Medicare study. Arthritis Res Ther 2012;14(4): R166.

3. Mekkes JR, Loots MA, Van Der Wal AC, et al. Causes, investigation and treatment of leg ulceration. Br J Dermatol 2003;148(3):388–401.

4. Labropoulos N, Manalo D, Patel NP, et al. Uncommon leg ulcers in the lower extremity. J Vasc Surg 2007;45(3):568–73.

5. Shanmugam VK, Angra D, Rahimi H, et al. Vasculitic and autoimmune wounds. J Vasc Surg Venous Lymphat Disord 2017;5(2):280–92.

6. Shanmugam VK, Schilling A, Germinario A, et al. Prevalence of immune disease in patients with wounds presenting to a tertiary wound healing centre. Int Wound J 2012;9(4):403–11.

7. Garwood CS, Kim PJ, Matai V, et al. The use of bovine collagen-glycosaminoglycan matrix for atypical lower extremity ulcers. Wounds 2016; 28(9):298–305.

8. Escandon J, Vivas AC, Tang J, et al. High mortality in patients with chronic wounds. Wound Repair Regen 2011;19:526–8.

9. Price P, Harding K. The impact of foot complications on health-related quality of life in patients with diabetes. J Cutan Med Surg 2000;4:45–50.

10. Li J, Chen J, Kirsner R. Pathophysiology of acute wound healing. Clin Dermatol 2007;25(1):9–18.

11. Broughton G 2nd, Janis JE, Attinger CE. The basic science of wound healing. Plast Reconstr Surg 2006;117(7 Suppl):12S–34S.
12. Shanmugam VK, Steen VD, Cupps TR. Lower extremity ulcers in connective tissue disease. Isr Med Assoc J 2008;10(7):534–6.
13. Rocca PV, Siegel LB, Cupps TR. The concomitant expression of vasculitis and coagulopathy: synergy for marked tissue ischemia. J Rheumatol 1994;21(3):556–60.
14. Braswell SF, Kostopoulos TC, Ortega-Loayza AG. Pathophysiology of pyoderma gangrenosum (PG) an updated review. J Am Acad Dermatol 2015;73(4):691–8.
15. Su WP, Davis MD, Weenig RH, et al. Pyoderma gangrenosum: clinicopathologic correlation and proposed diagnostic criteria. Int J Dermatol 2004;43(11):790–800.
16. Maverakis E, Ma C, Shinkai K, et al. Diagnostic criteria of ulcerative pyoderma gangrenosum: a Delphi consensus of international experts. JAMA Dermatol 2018;154(4):461–6.
17. London NJ, Donnelly R. ABC of arterial and venous disease. Ulcerated lower limb. BMJ 2000;320(7249):1589–91.
18. Kim PJ, Attinger CE, Steinberg JS, et al. Building a multidisciplinary hospital-based wound care center: nuts and bolts. Plast Reconstr Surg 2016;138(3 Suppl):241S–7S.
19. Gottrup F, Holstein P, Jørgensen B, et al. A new concept of a multidisciplinary wound healing center and a national expert function of wound healing. Arch Surg 2001;136(7):765–72.
20. Edwards ML. Hyperbaric oxygen therapy. Part 1: history of and principles. J Vet Emerg Crit Care (San Antonio) 2010;20(3):284–8.
21. Weaver LK, editor. Hyperbaric oxygen therapy indications. North Palm Beach (FL): Best Publishing Company; 2014. p. iii.
22. Thom SR. Hyperbaric oxygen therapy: its mechanisms and efficacy. Plast Reconstr Surg 2011;127(suppl):131S–41S.
23. Sheikh AY, Gibson JJ, Rollins MD, et al. Effect of hyperoxia on vascular endothelial growth factor levels in a wound model. Arch Surg 2000;135:1293–7.
24. Koomanachai P, Keel RA, Johnson-Arbor KK, et al. Linezolid penetration into wound tissue of two diabetic patients before and after hyperbaric oxygen therapy. Undersea Hyperb Med 2011;38(1):11–6.
25. Marx RE, Johnson RP. Problem wounds in oral and maxillofacial surgery: the role of hyperbaric oxygen. In: Davis JM, Hunt TK, editors. Problem wounds: the role of oxygen. New York: Elsevier; 1988. p. 65–125.
26. Li G, Hopkins RB, Levine MAH, et al. Relationship between hyperbaric oxygen therapy and quality of life in participants with chronic diabetic foot ulcers: data from a randomized controlled trial. Acta Diabetol 2017;54:823–31.
27. Mutluoglu M, Cakkalkurt A, Uzun G, et al. Topical oxygen for chronic wounds: a pro/con debate. J Am Coll Clin Wound Spec 2015;5:61–5.
28. UHMS position statement: topical oxygen for chronic wounds. Undersea Hyperb Med 2018;45(3):379–80.
29. Bakker K, Apelqvist J, Schaper NC. Practical guidelines on the management and prevention of the diabetic foot 2011. Diabetes Metab Res Rev 2012;28(suppl 1):225–31.
30. Centers for Medicare & Medicaid Services. National coverage determination (NCD) for hyperbaric oxygen therapy (20.29). 2017. Available at: CMS.gov; https://www.cms.gov/medicare-coverage-database/details/ncd-details.aspx?ncdid=12&ver=3. Accessed December 12, 2018.
31. Wagner FW. The diabetic foot. Orthopedics 1987;10(1):163–72.

32. Abidia A, Laden G, Kuhan G, et al. The role of hyperbaric oxygen therapy in ischaemic diabetic lower extremity ulcers: a double blind randomised-controlled trial. Eur J Vasc Endovasc Surg 2003;25:513–8.

33. Kaya A, Aydin F, Altay T. Can major amputation rates be decreased in diabetic foot ulcers with hyperbaric oxygen therapy? Int Orthop 2009;33:441–6.

34. Londahl M, Katzman P, Nilsson A, et al. Hyperbaric oxygen therapy facilitates healing of chronic foot ulcers in patients with diabetes. Diabetes Care 2010; 33(5):998–1003.

35. Duzgun AP, Satir HZ, Ozozan O, et al. Effect of hyperbaric oxygen therapy on healing of diabetic foot ulcers. J Foot Ankle Surg 2008;47(6):515–9.

36. Huang ET, Mansouri J, Murad MH, et al. A clinical practice guideline for the use of hyperbaric oxygen therapy in the treatment of diabetic foot ulcers. Undersea Hyperb Med 2015;42(3):205–47.

37. Margolis DJ, Gupta J, Hoffstad O, et al. Lack of effectiveness of hyperbaric oxygen therapy for the treatment of diabetic foot ulcer and the prevention of amputation. Diabetes Care 2013;36(7):1961–6.

38. Fedorko L, Bowen JM, Jones W, et al. Hyperbaric oxygen therapy does not reduce indications for amputation in patients with diabetes with nonhealing ulcers of the lower limb: a prospective, double-blind, randomized controlled clinical trial. Diabetes Care 2016;39(3):392–9.

39. Santema KT, Stoekenbroek RM, Koelemay MJW. Hyperbaric oxygen therapy in the treatment of ischemic lower extremity ulcers in patients with diabetes: results of the DAMO2CLES multicenter randomized clinical trial. Diabetes Care 2018; 41(1):112–9.

40. Sheffield PJ, Desautels DA. Hyperbaric and hypobaric chamber fires: a 73-year analysis. Undersea Hyperb Med 1997;24(3):153–64.

41. National Fire Protection Agency. Chapter 14: hyperbaric facilities. In: NFPA 99 2015 edition health care facilities code. Quincy (MA): National Fire Protection Agency; 2015. p. 105–17.